COMING
of
AGE

Lois Mowday Rabey

OLIVER
NELSON

THOMAS NELSON PUBLISHERS

Nashville • Atlanta • London • Vancouver

TO

ANN REED

*She aged so gracefully that
those of us who knew her
were not even aware that she
was getting any older.*

Published in Nashville, Tennessee, by Thomas Nelson, Inc., Publishers, and
distributed in Canada by Word Communications, Ltd., Richmond, British
Columbia.

The Bible version used in this publication is THE NEW KING JAMES
VERSION. Copyright © 1979, 1980, 1982, 1990, Thomas Nelson, Inc.,
Publishers.

Library of Congress Cataloging-in-Publication Data

Rabey, Lois Mowday.
    Coming of age / Lois Mowday Rabey.
        p.   m.
    Includes bibliographical references and index.
    ISBN 0-7852-8145-2
    1. Menopause—Popular works.   2. Middle aged women—Psychology.
    I. Title.
RG186.R33   1995   94-44027
612.6'65—dc20   CIP

Printed in the United States of America.

1 2 3 4 5 6—00 99 98 97 96 95

CONTENTS

....

*A*CKNOWLEDGMENTS
....

There are always so many people to thank for helping in the process of completing a book, from those who do the nitty-gritty work of editing to the behind-the-scenes prayer supporters. The following are special *thank you's* to just a few of those people.

- To the women in the focus groups, who were all a delight. Thank you for being open, honest, and so much fun. To the women who set up and hosted these group interviews, you made the research go so smoothly that I hated to see it end.

- To Willy Wooten and your wonderful group of men who met to talk, you surprised me and changed my mind about how many men think about menopause.

- To Helen Ricles and the staff of The Women's Mid-life Health Center, Swedish Medical Center, who were so informative and encouraging.

- To Marie Campbell for helping me establish a personal exercise program for the first time in my life. You were a great encouragement and source of valuable information.

• To the many friends who prayed and called to see how I was doing at various stages of this project. A special thank you to four women who are faithful in their concern for me: Loretta Fellhauer, Claudette Gomez, Joanne Huddleson, and Susan Pannell. You are terrific!

• To Victor Oliver for continuing to be my friend, publisher, and advisor. And to Rose Marie for many helpful conversations when Victor was out of the office.

• To Lisa and Chadd, Lara and Craig for keeping my spirits up in all circumstances. I love you all and am so blessed to have such supportive daughters and sons-in-law.

• To my husband, Steve, who stayed up late and worked weekends to edit this manuscript. I know the subject matter was not your usual area of interest, but you were great. I value your opinion above all others.

• And finally, to the staff of Valley View Health Care Center, Canon City, Colorado, for so wonderfully taking care of my father. If he had not been in such good hands, I would not have been able to complete this project.

*I*NTRODUCTION

I am neither shy nor easily embarrassed. In fact, sometimes I cause others to blush because of my feisty relational style. People never need wonder what I am thinking, for I will tell them if they hang around longer than thirty seconds.

But a few months ago I found myself in an unusual situation. My husband, Steve, and I went to visit The Tattered Cover, a bookstore in Denver. It is a four-story paradise of volume-filled shelves, overstuffed chairs, dark wood accoutrements, and an eclectic clientele.

As we approached the front door, I realized I was feeling anxious. I stopped and pulled Steve out of the way of the steady stream of ingoing customers.

"I want you to get a book for me," I said in a low tone.

He looked puzzled.

"I don't want to ask for it myself, and I don't want to go up and pay for it myself."

Steve scrunched his eyebrows together until lines in his forehead appeared.

"Why?" he finally managed to ask.

"I don't want anyone to know," I said, glancing over my shoulder like a character in a French spy novel.

"Lois, what are you talking about?"

"I want Gail Sheehy's book *Silent Passage,* about—you know—uh—women my age. Actually, it's about women a little older than I am—you know, fifty or so—but I *am* almost there and I feel—*you know.*"

"No, I don't know," he said, "and I think it's okay for you to ask for it yourself."

Terror! He wasn't going to cooperate. He had slipped from my grasp and was through the revolving doors and into the store before I could plead my case.

"Steve!" I called as I ran to catch up with him. "Wait. You have to help me. Just get the book for me and that will be the end of it."

"The end of what?" he turned and asked with the same puzzled look on his face.

He doesn't know, I thought. *He thinks that I'm my usual assertive self: confident and unafraid. I haven't told him that I am embarrassed to be old enough to need to read a book about women "that age."*

"Oh, never mind," I said out loud.

Steve looked relieved. We decided to meet by the first floor checkout desk in an hour, and Steve headed for the stairs. But I stood motionless by the front door, feeling confused. I was surprised at myself. I had to have that book, but I was actually sweating over the prospect of someone seeing me buy it. There was some painful kind of recognition taking place that I was admitting to the world what the world already knew: Women face significant and sometimes distressing changes between the ages of forty and fifty-five due to the process of menopause, and I (youthful, active, energetic) had reached the stage where I was going through some of these changes. I had been thinking that if I didn't admit to some of the discomfort I was experiencing, no one would think that I was aging. How silly! The evidence was all there: My hair was gray; my children were grown; I was about to become a grandmother; my skin showed the unmistakable signs of weathering.

The only one I was kidding was myself. To admit that I wanted some advice on this subject did not reveal any revolutionary secret to anyone but me. I was shocked at my own resistance to the inevitable. My life had included several dramatic changes that I always handled with a degree of calm. Now, here I was in a crowded bookstore, sweating and feeling nervous over buying a book.

My desire for the book motivated me enough to climb the stairs to the second floor. But in a store that carries over 225,000 titles, finding the general topic of interest alone is a challenge. I knew that I wanted the area devoted to women's studies, but I couldn't find it. Panic surfaced as I realized anew I would have to ask for help.

How old am I? I scolded myself, feeling thirteen.

I finally found a workstation with two female salesclerks at the computer terminals. I didn't want a man even to hear me ask for the book. I quietly asked one of the women if they had the book *Silent Passage*. She immediately headed across the room with me in tow like a bashful child.

The women's section covered seven long shelves. I quickly picked up *Silent Passage* and moved away from the telltale area. As I continued to browse through the rest of the bookstore, I kept my arm tightly around the book so that no one could see the title. An hour later, when Steve and I met at the checkout counter, I quickly handed him the book. He took it without question and put it with his stack of purchases. I lingered around the fiction section until he was done. We left, and my discomfort ended. Temporarily.

Only a few weeks later, I began to have the symptoms that were mentioned in Sheehy's book: anxiety, memory loss, mood swings. And just like the title says, I remained silent. But the isolation made me feel crazy. Why did I not hear other women talking about these things? I knew I couldn't be the only one in my circle of friends who was feeling this way. I broke the silence and began to ask other women my age if they were experiencing any of these strange new interruptions to normalcy.

"Yes, yes!" one after another excitedly replied, relieved not to be alone.

Venturing into conversations with these women led to the writing of this book. I interviewed over one hundred women and heard at least that many variations of the way women handle moving through the mid-life years. These women talked about menopause and its impact on all areas of their lives—thinking, decisions, relationships.

I also talked with some men about their feelings as their wives face menopause. The stories of these men and women, and my own, are woven through this book. (The names have been changed but the stories are related as they were told.) Some of them are funny, some tragic, each showing how unique and personal each episode of menopause is.

Perhaps you are thinking, *Menopause? What's the big deal? I'll simply proceed the way I always have.*

That was my attitude. I had never even thought seriously about menopause because I didn't know that much about it. I knew that I didn't intend to grow old the way I had seen some women do. I told myself for years that I simply would not gain weight, would not become an emotional basketcase, and would not be fazed by the life changes that would occur. My faith in God's provision and my moxie would carry me through.

Then one day, as I dissolved one time too many in a puddle of tears, I had to admit that my old ways of coping were not enough to get me through this new, unique experience. Something was missing. I began to question my ability to appropriate my faith and flogged myself for falling short of peaceful calm or not rising above my circumstances.

I had always been able to draw on spiritual realities to overcome anything, including the death of my first husband. But now I felt disconnected from God when something as simple as an emotional low occurred. I prayed and paced and panicked and finally realized that I needed information, encouragement, and help.

God was there in the panic, is here now, and will be here always. Many of the women I interviewed experienced the same spiritual self-doubt as they stumbled through these years of disruption. Their stories, and mine, are a testimony to the steadfastness of God. He accepts us in our frustration, our doubt, our learning, and our changes. And as in all things, He uses it to our good.

I still cannot believe I am in my late forties. It seems like my thirty-year high school reunion last fall should have been my ten-year reunion. When I watch football games I still feel like the cheerleader I once was so long ago. I hold a baby and picture my own children, who are now in their twenties, as infants. I visit my dad in the nursing home where he lives and am shocked to see that I am the parent-figure and he is like a child.

I accept where I am in this new coming of age. I try to think and act like a mature woman. But sometimes— inside, unseen, unheard—I scream to myself, *I'm too young to be this old!*

CHAPTER 1

WHAT IS HAPPENING TO ME?

*T*echnically speaking, menopause is the cessation of a woman's menstrual cycle, occurring sometime between the ages of forty and fifty-five. But the internal changes that culminate in this event begin many years earlier. These internal changes can produce symptoms that appear one month and may not return until many months later. The woman may be alarmed by the symptom and surprised to find out it is related to menopause.

That's what happened to me.

Surprised and Afraid

I was forty-three years old, a bride again of four months, and feeling great. I was looking forward to visiting my husband's hometown in Ohio. It was a combination work and pleasure trip as I was to speak on Sunday morning in the church where he had accepted Christ years ago.

We arrived Friday, on a beautiful fall afternoon. The trees had just begun to change colors and the air had a slight tinge of chilliness. We enjoyed a few hours of nostalgia as we drove around looking at the places Steve had lived, the high school and college he had attended, and his favorite haunts. That night we joined his family for a leisurely dinner at their favorite restaurant. All indications were that we had a relaxing weekend ahead of us.

In the middle of the night, I woke up feeling bloated and slightly uncomfortable. I went to the bathroom and was surprised to find that I was bleeding heavily. My period, always uneventful and easy, should have been almost over. By morning, I had been up several more times and continued to be perplexed by the heavy bleeding. Otherwise, I felt fine: no cramps, no other symptoms at all.

We began our day of scheduled visiting with a number of Steve's friends. I assumed I would be fine so long as I made a rest room stop every hour or so. But by three o'clock that afternoon, I couldn't make it more than ten alarming minutes. Embarrassed in front of strangers, I had to excuse myself to go to the bathroom continually. Finally, I told Steve that I was really a little scared and thought I should go to a twenty-four-hour emergency medical office. There was no way I could speak the next day if the bleeding continued at this rate.

On the way to the clinic, I was afraid and confused. I had never had any trouble whatsoever with my period. The only thing I knew about abnormal bleeding was that it was one of the symptoms of cancer. I envisioned a huge tumor in my body about to explode. I felt no physical pain, but emotionally, I was in agony.

We arrived at the clinic, and I felt a measure of relief in knowing help was at hand. The receptionist put me in a room to see the doctor as soon as I had filled out the registration information. I was embarrassed at the thought of being examined by a stranger when I was such a mess. The nurse was very sympathetic. "Don't worry," she said kindly, "the doctor sees a number of women in similar emergencies."

Similar to what? I asked myself. I had never heard any woman say anything about this kind of episode.

The doctor was very pleasant and reassuring. He said the heavy bleeding was probably a hormonal imbalance related to my age. I thought to myself, *My age? What about my age?* I didn't ask him what he meant. I just wanted him to fix whatever this was.

He gave me a hormone shot and told me to see my own doctor as soon as I got home. I promised him that I would and persisted in getting *him* to promise *me* that I would not be embarrassed when I stood in front of a church full of people the next morning. He promised.

"You'll dry up like a desert in an hour or so," he said.

I was exhausted. Steve and I canceled our evening plans and went back to our hotel. We ate in the room and watched television. My thoughts were preoccupied with making it through my speaking engagement the next morning and the plane ride home that afternoon.

But the doctor was right. My body reacted to the shot in the manner of a gushing faucet that has been suddenly turned off. The bleeding stopped completely. It wasn't until we were on the plane on the way home that I thought again about what had caused the bleeding. It couldn't be related to menopause, because that only had to do with hot flashes and the cessation of bleeding. Besides, menopause happened to older women, not to me at the age of forty-three. I was worried that the bleeding was a sign of cancer.

I called my doctor first thing Monday morning. Tuesday morning I was in her office telling her of my harrowing experience. Since the bleeding had been so heavy, she suggested one of two things: a biopsy to rule out cancer or a D and C (dilatation and curettage—scraping of the uterus), not only to rule out cancer but also to prevent future similar episodes. I tend to make quick decisions and remained in character that day.

"Let's go for the D and C and get this over with," I said assertively, confident that this temporary problem would be over. The doctor thought I would be fine to have the procedure done in her office with local anesthesia.

My husband and I arrived at the doctor's office on the appointed morning. By that time, I had grown nervous about the procedure. The day before, I had talked with a girlfriend who had had a D and C and she swore she would never have one again without anesthesia that knocked her completely out. I decided to keep my appointment to have it done in the doctor's office and stay awake, but her words lingered in my mind.

I was given a shot to calm me and make me sleepy. I was barely awake. The procedure was a little uncomfortable but not really painful. My perception of time blurred completely. When it was over, I had to be led to the car by my husband and I immediately fell asleep on the ride home. There was little else in the way of inconvenience for me (though that is not always the case, as will be seen in the following chapters).

The D and C revealed no evidence of cancer. The diagnosis was hormonal changes. It may be hard to believe that I didn't ask any further questions. But at the time I accepted this pronouncement to mean my hormones were fluctuating and no other symptoms would occur. Just in case another episode of bleeding did occur, my doctor prescribed birth control pills, which contain hormones, to have on hand. Taking one or two of them would stop any unexpected bleeding.*

Life went back to normal and I almost forgot the whole incident. The bleeding, which I now know was hemorrhaging, happened again about a year later. This time I had the birth control pills with me. Once again I was out of town for a speaking engagement, so when I returned home I called my doctor. This time she did a biopsy instead of a D and C. (A biopsy examines tissue to rule out cancer but does nothing to prevent further bleeding.) Again, thankfully, no cancer. The diagnosis: hormonal.

Unlike my experience with the D and C, the biopsy actually caused more bleeding. This, too, is normal, but it was nonetheless disconcerting. I became apprehensive about future episodes of unexpected hemorrhaging and carried tampons with me all the time, along with the magic pills that would shut the spigot off. There were three more incidents in four years and all three occurred when I was traveling. And I learned that this is a normal, early symptom of menopause.

In the years since that first sign, I have learned to live with a general sense of watchfulness. Other symptoms have kicked in, including anxiety attacks, dizziness, and forgetfulness, all of which will be discussed in later chapters. There is no pattern or consistency with any of these interruptions to normal life. Anytime, anywhere, I can start bleeding, sweating, feeling dizzy, or emoting dramatically.

This probably doesn't sound like good news! But by being informed and prepared for what is to come, much

---

*Warning: Always consult carefully with your doctor. If there is a possibility that you are pregnant when bleeding occurs, taking medications with hormones is dangerous.

of the fear and uncertainty of the beginning phases of menopause can be alleviated.

The Beginning of a Process

The first symptoms of menopause signal the beginning of a process that can last for several years.

In the book *Managing Your Menopause,* Dr. Wulf Utian and Ruth S. Jacobowitz define the word that is used to describe this entire process.

> The word "climacteric" comes from the Greek and means "critical time." Sometime during this so-called critical time, (generally a ten-year span between the ages of forty-five and fifty-five) your last period will occur—usually when you're around the age of fifty. But changes are happening long before that time, and beginning in your thirties, you may not only notice them but you can do something about them.[1]

The process unfolds this way:

1. Sometime during the age range of the thirties, forties, or fifties, a woman's body begins to produce less estrogen than it has been since the onset of menstruation.
2. The levels of estrogen production in the body fluctuate over a period of years, called the *climacteric.*
3. These fluctuating levels of estrogen result in changes that manifest themselves in numerous symptoms. (Section 2 deals extensively with symptoms.)
4. Eventually the body stops producing estrogen completely and menstruation occurs for the last time. This event is called *menopause.*

Often the word *menopause* is used to refer to the entire process of the climacteric. That is how the process will be defined in this book.

Understanding menopause and how to respond to it can help a woman move through the process more smoothly than a woman who begins with little warning or knowledge. But why don't women know more about this process?

Why Are We So Silent?

My mother was from the old school. You know, the one that touted the doctrine: *You should never talk about religion, politics, or sex.* I never questioned her but accepted that these subjects were off-limits. While religion and politics filtered into our dinnertime conversations occasionally, s-e-x *never* did.

My parents' involvement in my sex education consisted of my mother clandestinely giving me a book when I was twelve and telling me to read it. I remember it being excessively technical and boring, with no pictures or sketches, which was disappointing. Of course, the other kids at school had long ago told me about "the birds and the bees." So, after about a week I handed the book back to my mother without a word. She took it and that was that.

When I was growing up, my mother never mentioned menopause. It might be assumed that as one's own mother entered this life passage, a daughter would hear (or overhear) what was happening. I did not. My mother was rushed to the hospital one morning when I was ten years old. She was forty-six and had some sudden secret something happen in the middle of the night. My father took her to the hospital and I stayed home with my grandmother, who helped keep the secret. When my father came home later that day, he told me she had had a hysterectomy and would be home soon. I didn't know what a hysterectomy was and didn't ask. I was simply glad when she came home and all was well again.

Both my mother and father treated any sexual subjects as shameful. The fact that menopause involves a woman's sex organs would have been enough to keep them silent.

Many women now over the age of forty grew up in households similar to mine. Their parents did not talk about sex and their mothers did not talk about their menopause when it occurred. Some of these women have since asked their mothers about this taboo topic. The ones whose mothers talked freely described symptoms just like those their daughters are experiencing today. They suffered in silence.

Our mothers' silence may be easier to understand after a look at how menopausal women have been portrayed in recent history.

The Menopausal Woman: Hysterical and Self-indulgent

At the beginning of the twentieth century, many people (men *and* women) thought that menopause equaled insanity. Menopausal women were described as hysterical females who were oversexed, self-indulgent, and subject to madness.

One of the popular books of the day was *The Dangerous Age*, a novel by Karin Michaelis published in 1911. The central character, Elsie Lindtner, divorces her husband and runs away with a younger man. This behavior is attributed to her mad state as a result of her age.

Lois Banner describes Elsie and her friends in her book *In Full Flower*.

As the novel progresses, most of Lindtner's middle-aged women friends suffer emotional breakdowns. Some alternate between mania and depression; some leave their husbands. Some become obsessive; one woman cleans her house over and over again. Another is institutionalized and treated surgically.[2]

This view was so prevalent in the early 1900s that it was reflected in the name chosen for the surgery common to women between the ages of forty and fifty: *hysterectomy*. Banner explains how this word came into existence:

> Michaelis's presentation of menopause as producing insanity resonated in the views of many gynecologists. Drawing on misperceptions standard for centuries, many gynecologists posited a direct linkage between the uterus and the brain. (Such a belief would result in the term "hysterectomy" for the removal of the uterus and ovaries, referencing the mental condition of hysteria and its presumed connection to female reproductive organs.) And such beliefs were extended to aging women.[3]

Not everyone agreed with this negative picture of menopausal women. In 1912, the opposite image was popularized in the book *Woman's Share in Social Culture* by Anna Garlin Spencer. Banner describes this view: "Spencer drew from contemporary evidence that women lived longer than men and were more vital in older years to assert that menopause afforded women a 'second youth.'"[4]

These two conflicting views of menopausal women have continued to cause confusion. Banner continues, "The first opinion has been that menopause is an illness bringing a breakdown of body and mind. The second has been that menopause initiates a time of strength for women. . . ."[5]

By the 1930s and 1940s, it seemed as if the first opinion was winning the popularity poll. Growing numbers of women were being diagnosed as insane due to menopause. Hospitals had whole sections for mentally disturbed, menopausal women.

It is easy to understand why my mother and other women her age would have decided to keep quiet about any menopausal symptoms they were experiencing. They could have found themselves institutionalized as a result of speaking out.

What Does the Bible Say?

Menopause is not mentioned directly in the Bible, but there are two examples of women who bore children after they were no longer of childbearing age: Sarah in the Old Testament and Elizabeth in the New Testament.

In the Old Testament, we read, "Now Abraham and Sarah were old, well advanced in age; and Sarah had passed the age of childbearing" (Gen. 18:11). God intervened and Sarah gave birth to Isaac.

In the New Testament, Elizabeth is also past childbearing age. Her husband, Zacharias, is visited by an angel who tells him that he and Elizabeth will have a son. Zacharias replies, "How shall I know this? For I am an old man, and my wife is well advanced in years" (Luke 1:18).

These passages are silent with regard to menopause except to show that God chose to intervene in the lives of both these women and give them children even after they were old. But while the Bible is silent about menopause, it has much to say about age.

When my daughter Lara was in the sixth grade, she had to find a Bible verse that described her mother. At the end of the school day she proudly brought me home the paper with her verse describing me. "The silver-haired head is a crown of glory, if it is found in the way of righteousness" (Prov. 16:31).

I was thirty-eight years old at the time, but my hair was very gray (I have always preferred to call it *white*). Lara beamed up at me as I read her paper. I smiled, hugged her, and thanked her for thinking of me as righteous, evidenced in part by my silver crown.

It was a mixed blessing: My daughter admired me but described me as aged. The incident made me realize, however, that the Bible does have some positive things to say about aging. Older people are presented as possessing wisdom worthy of respect:

> Wisdom is with aged men, And with length of days, understanding (Job 12:12).

> You shall rise before the gray headed and honor the presence of an old man, and fear your God: I am the LORD (Lev. 19:32).

Scripture also acknowledges declining health in old age.

> Now the eyes of Israel were dim with age, so that he could not see (Gen. 48:10).

> Do not cast me off in the time of old age; Do not forsake me when my strength fails (Ps. 71:9).

Perhaps the most well-known biblical text that describes a godly woman is Proverbs 31. This passage focuses on the character of a wise woman, not her physical condition. It lifts up the qualities of virtue, industriousness, wisdom, kindness, and fear of the Lord.

The Bible paints a picture that defines women without reference to menopause and uplifts both men and women who attain an old age. But current society has not pursued the same ideals.

A Culture Obsessed with Youth

America worships the cult of youth. The cosmetic industry is a prime example of turning that worship into a money-making endeavor. One of the target markets for cosmetic companies is the menopausal woman. There are anti-aging products for every body part, with advertisements claiming miraculous results from the daily use of these gold-priced wonder creams.

A few years ago I ordered a body lotion from a store in Florida beause the particular product line is not sold in Colorado. The lotion was for general use, anywhere on the body.

When the package arrived in the mail, it contained an additional *fourteen* different samples of anti-aging potions. There was a cream for the eyes, nose, mouth, elbows, hands, feet, thighs, legs, and "special" creams to boot. Evidently each cream knew to work if it was correctly applied to the designated body part, but not on any other part. Heaven forbid that you mix up your eye cream with your thigh cream. No telling what would happen!

I sadly confess that I have tried a number of these panaceas for aging. I have now faced the stark reality that, of course, they don't work. Why have I wasted so much money on such foolishness? Because I have bought the American dream that youth is the only form of acceptable beauty and swallowed the cosmetic companies' claims of regaining a youthful appearance by using a wonder cream. Intellectually I know that this is not true, but it is difficult to dash the hope of looking forever young.

Attitudes Are Changing

Fortunately, I am changing my mind and am beginning to give up my quest for the fountain of youth in a bottle. In the writing of this book I met the most engaging women who unashamedly accept the physical results of aging with style. They don't worry about wrinkles or a little weight. They take care of themselves physically but operate on the truth that beauty is more than skin deep. Advertising may be targeting older women with the promise of looking younger, but many older women are focusing on far more fulfilling arenas. They are trying to improve in areas of life where they can learn and grow instead of trying to be something they are not.

Evidence of changing attitudes is also being seen in the area of women's health. Menopausal women are the subject of new health initiatives that are seeking to answer problems specifically related to these women. The shift in demographics in this country is undoubtedly dictating some of this increased attention. Gayle Sand in her book *Is It Hot in Here or Is It Me?* says, "The climacteric has become the focus of talk shows and other public forums for two important reasons: First, 42 million women in this year alone will be experiencing the climacteric; second, the baby boomers are growing up."[6]

Health magazine reports: "Over the next decade, 21

million women of the baby boom generation will enter menopause."[7]

Women's mid-life medical clinics are popping up across the country, and increased amounts of money are being put into research. *Vogue* magazine reported:

> Two studies are under way to help answer the [hormone] question. The National Institute of Health has launched the Post-Menopausal Estrogen/Progestin Interventions Trial (PEPI). At Johns Hopkins and six other centers, it will compare women taking estrogen alone with those also taking different types of progestin. The larger Women's Health Initiative will assess long-term risks and benefits in 70,000 postmenopausal women.[8]

So while our culture continues to grapple with what is beautiful and what is not, millions of women are getting older and trying to answer more significant health questions. Effective and safe treatment for menopause is high on the list of priorities.

Beauty is beginning to be equated more with health than with youth among women today. Some men may still define beauty by the eye, but women are becoming more interested in defining beauty by how well they feel. They are less obsessed with being bone thin and more concerned with preserving bone density.

Talking About Menopause

Just a few months ago, I was in Palm Springs, California, to speak at a conference. I drove in from San Diego where I had been visiting my daughters. The drive didn't take me as long as I anticipated, so I stopped at an outlet mall to browse through the stores. I felt good and was particularly proud of myself for having exercised that morning. I was sticking to my goal of exercising, even on the road.

One jewelry store displayed enticing signs that announced discounts of 40 percent to 60 percent off each purchase. I picked out some earrings for myself and my daughters and went to the counter. The clerk, a woman about my age, smiled and rang up the items with the discounts. Then she said brightly, "And you get an additional ten percent off!"

"Great!" I smiled back. "How come?"

She pointed to a sign on the wall behind her.

TUESDAY IS SENIOR DISCOUNT DAY—
ADDITIONAL 10% OFF

I was shocked. My heart started to race, and I had to stifle the urge to punch this friendly lady right in the mouth. Senior Discount! I was not even forty-nine yet. How dare she!

That did it for shopping that day. I took my old, exercised body and slinked to my rental car. The four-door Lincoln *did* look old-lady-ish. I wanted to shout that I had a car rental discount coupon, not based on age, for a two-level upgrade. I really should have been driving a Mustang.

The clerk in the store hadn't meant to insult me. She was simply giving me an added discount on merchandise. But I was wounded and outraged. And I realized how sensitive I would need to be if I were to approach women for interviews for a book on menopause.

I was pleasantly surprised. The first women I talked to were so enthusiastic, I decided to try another idea. I asked women if they would be willing to be interviewed in focus groups of approximately the same age range.

The first group met during lunchtime (they all worked). I was amazed at the openness. Nobody wanted to stop at the end of the hour. I found myself greatly encouraged and less anxious about some of my own symptoms and feelings. Other women had experienced the same things. They were able to laugh, talk, offer suggestions. The atmosphere was warm and relaxing, exactly the opposite of what I had anticipated.

After that first one all the groups met in women's homes. When the research was completed, a few of the groups even decided to continue to meet as support groups. The setting was safe, and the stories of other women comforting.

The silence seems to be over and women are ready to talk. These women want other women to go through menopause with more information and less mystery than they brought with them.

CHAPTER 2

HOT AND COLD
AND
ALL SHOOK UP

*O*ne of the hallmarks of menopause is the variety and unpredictability of symptoms. Some women experience very few symptoms, others experience them all—sometimes at the same time.

Even with this variability, hot flashes and night sweats are two of the most common symptoms of menopause, with an estimated 75 to 85 percent of menopausal women suffering from them. They are actually the same symptom, differentiated by when they occur. *Night sweats* happen in the middle of the night, interrupting sleep. *Hot flashes* happen during waking hours. Both last longer than an instant but usually not more than five minutes. The most definitive element of these symptoms is their unpredictability.

Drs. Sharon and David Sneed describe hot flashes this way in their book *Prime Time*. "The flushes are extremely unpredictable, occurring with varying frequency, intensity, and duration. They are usually described as a sudden, uncomfortable feeling of intense warmth in the face, neck, and chest."[1]

Hot flashes and night sweats are related to decreasing

levels of estrogen in the body, but little is known as to why a drop in estrogen sets off these reactions. Utian and Jacobowitz summarize current knowledge:

> What we do know, however, is that when estrogen pro-
> duction drops abruptly during the perimenopause [the
> years prior to the cessation of a woman's period], there
> is a change in the brain's chemistry that affects the tem-
> perature control center in the hypothalamus. The result
> is a decrease in the body's core temperature set point
> that triggers dilation of the blood vessels of the skin and
> sweating as the body attempts to reset its thermostat.[2]

Although hot flashes are not dangerous, they can be embarrassing. Others may not seem to notice a woman's dripping appearance anywhere near as much as the woman thinks they do, but a woman suffering a hot flash feels exposed.

And a lack of notice does not mean that a woman is exaggerating the degree of heat she feels and the amount of perspiration her body is producing. Perhaps others who are with a woman experiencing a hot flash don't notice for two reasons: (1) We are so self-absorbed we don't look carefully at others, and (2) people per-spire at all ages. This is considered a rather normal body function and draws little attention.

Hot flashes are certainly a disturbing symptom of menopause. They reinforce a sense of being out of con-trol over your own body and disrupt normal life. But they don't last forever—it just seems like they will.

Hot Flash Stories

I have experienced only one bona fide hot flash. When it hit there was no premonition of impending calamity. Life was going along as usual. I was in my early forties and felt great. My plan to age without evidence was working.

I had been on a speaking trip to the East Coast and was coming back home by way of Chicago. I took advantage of the layover to visit a girlfriend. She and I were eating a wonderfully elegant dinner in a well-known downtown restaurant. I was just digging into a decadent chocolate-chocolate dessert when *it* happened. Sweat started to pour out of my skin like a spigot turned on full throttle. I gasped with fear and the need for air. I pulled the collar of my blouse away from my neck and felt a rush of tropical steam blast my face. My friend was unaware of my hysteria, her attention fully given to her own chocolate-chocolate dessert.

Panic seized me as I realized that this breaking of some hidden reservoir was not stopping. I slammed the palms of my hands against the edge of the table and bolted without explanation to my friend. The first breath of relief came when I burst out the front door of the restaurant into the middle of the busy Chicago sidewalk. The doorman evidently had seen this kind of behavior before, for he simply smiled politely as I hung onto the awning pole sucking in the cold night air.

I was still standing there drawing in air and spurting out steam when my confused friend found me.

"What is happening?" she asked with puzzled concern.

"I am so *hot*!" I yelled. I could breathe now, but residual heat was still seeping out of my shaking body.

My friend looked at me with an expression of dismay as she shivered in the winter night cold. I was only forty-two, but she was a mere youth of thirty. I didn't realize that I had experienced a hot flash; she didn't even know what a hot flash was.

I am grateful (though mystified as to why) that I have not experienced that particular pandemonium again. Most women who suffer from hot flashes are not so blessed. Their first one is usually followed by an unpredictable series of body-thermostat failures.

Marge is a beautiful blond in her late forties who loves to dress in luscious silk dresses. She is meticulous—never a wrinkle, certainly never a perspiration stain. Her first hot flash happened in church on Easter.

"We were sitting near the front, of course," she told the group of women gathered to talk about menopause.

"I had on a pale blue silk dress and all of a sudden, I was sweating. My dress started to stick to my skin—everywhere! My hair was stuck to my head. I looked like someone had poured a bucket of water over me. It was awful. There was nowhere to go, no way to sneak out. I was drenched from the skin out," she insisted, able to smile now at the recollection.

Betty spoke up. She said she didn't know if she had ever had a hot flash or not. The response was unanimous.

"If you don't know, then you haven't had one."

A hot flash is far more than a feeling of being very hot. I lived in Florida for thirteen years and was very hot most of the time. Just going from an air-conditioned house to an air-conditioned car was enough time, in sultry south Florida heat, for your whole body to break out in a sweat. But as hot as that experience was, it is not like a hot flash.

Perspiration as a result of the weather is the body's response to an external change. In a hot flash the body is responding to an internal change. The heat starts deep inside and surges through the body, finally exploding through the pores of the skin. The feeling is one of being cooked all the way through. It is common to be consumed by a need for cool air and panicked at the suddenness and intensity of what is happening.

Some women respond in dramatic ways, as Ann shared with her group.

"I have a friend who was at a party—crowded, hot, stuffy—and had such a bad hot flash that she ran into the bathroom and ripped off her clothes." Ann's friend spent several minutes there naked, trying to compose herself. After cooling down, she put her soggy clothes back on, combed her damp hair, and rejoined the party.

Carol had hot flashes that worsened when she was caring for her sick father. "The stress was incredible. My body went nuts. Things got better after I was out from under so much stress."

Allison said that the thing she hated most about her hot flashes was the blinding sensation and dizziness that preceded them.

"I was at lunch with a woman I had just met. It was a business lunch, so I wanted to be fairly coherent. We were sitting at the table talking when everything dimmed. I had this moment of dizziness and knew what was coming. My vision cleared quickly but then the water started to pour. I took my suit jacket off, hoping she didn't notice why. The dizziness also was gone almost right away, but the sweat just wouldn't quit. My colleague graciously didn't comment. How could she have missed my sudden drenched appearance?"

A Bedtime Tale

All of these women experienced numerous hot flashes over varying periods of time. Many of them

spent sleepless nights because the drenchings also occurred in the dark.

Amy lives in the air-conditioned comfort of her lovely
Florida home. As she entered her mid-forties she started
to experience hot flashes during the day and night
sweats during the night. She kept lowering the thermo-
stat, but that didn't help. Her husband complained that
he was freezing to death at night under a pile of blankets
while she was burning up with no covers at all. She slept
in absorbent cotton nightgowns as recommended, but
she still was drenched night after night.

Barbara's husband actually had leg pains that he felt
were brought on by the temperature in the bedroom.
Kim's problem was exhaustion. "The night sweats keep
me awake most of the night," she said.

Suggestions for Survival

Many women find great relief from hot flashes and
night sweats by taking hormone replacement therapy
(HRT). Because these symptoms occur as a result of
decreases in estrogen, the increased estrogen in HRT
often solves the problem.

Many women who have tried natural remedies for relief of hot flashes have found relief by taking vitamin E.
The dosage varies with the woman, but the range is
usually between 400 IU to 1200 IU, taken one to three
times a day. Women with liver disease should check with
their doctors before taking vitamin E.

There are some indications that hot flashes and night
sweats may also be caused by a blood-sugar imbalance.

In Linda Ojeda's book *Menopause Without Medicine,*
she points out this correlation between women who experience hot flashes and the existence of a blood-sugar
imbalance, or hypoglycemia. She suggests, "If your first

menopausal symptom is a hot flash, consider: How many of the known triggers of both hot flashes and hypoglycemia—caffeine, alcohol, heavily spiced foods, sugar, and so on—are a normal part of your diet?"[3]

The women interviewed in the focus groups confirmed that hot flashes and night sweats are highly individualistic symptoms, and successful therapies are equally individualistic. Some women found almost immediate relief with HRT. Others noticed a change simply with increased dosages of vitamin E. Controlled diets helped others. And for some, nothing seemed to help.

If hot flashes and night sweats are relentless, even after using several different therapies, living with them is the only alternative. Here is some practical advice from women who have been in this unpredictable predicament.

- Wear nightgowns and underwear made of 100 percent cotton instead of nylon or other nonabsorbent material.
- If you are in an enclosed place like an office building when a hot flash occurs, get some fresh air as soon as possible. Excuse yourself and go outside for a few moments.
- Keep a cool glass of water handy and sip on it. This won't prevent a hot flash but can help to cool down the body.
- If you are going to be away from home all day, carry a change of underwear. At least when the hot flash ends, you can go and change into something dry. Some women even keep an extra blouse with them.
- If a hot flash occurs while you are around other people, slip off by yourself for a few moments and simply relax. Breathe deeply and slowly, take a drink of

water, and give your body an opportunity to calm down.

Irregular Periods

I have carried a daily planner for some twenty years. Without it, I don't know where I am or where I am supposed to be. In the front section with the month-at-a-glance, I have always put a lightly penciled circle around the date of my next expected period. I had never been off by more than two days in all those years until a year ago. I still pencil in those circles, but I use an eraser much more often now!

Sooner or later all women stop having periods, but it is uncommon for them to stop abruptly, neatly, or in a predictable pattern. It is much more common for women to have irregular periods before complete cessation occurs.

Missed periods are no cause for alarm, except for the possibility of an unexpected pregnancy. (Of all the women interviewed, none of them had an unexpected pregnancy during the process of menopause.) In general, a woman is considered to have completed menopause, and no longer be able to conceive a child, after her period has ceased for a year. But pregnancy can still occur during this unpredictable time. If you do not want a child at this stage of life, be sure to practice birth control of some kind until your doctor has declared you past your reproductive years. This can be determined by a simple blood test that registers hormone levels.

Increased bleeding is another story. This can be dangerous and demands immediate attention. Frequent bleeding takes several forms: spotting, more frequent periods, bleeding between regular periods, heavier and/or longer periods, and hemorrhaging.

In *Menopause and the Years Ahead,* Mary Beard and Lindsay Curtis explain what is happening when bleeding—spotting to hemorrhaging—occurs during menopause:

> Spotting is common during menopause because of decreasing estrogen production by the ovaries. When ovulation fails to occur because of the diminishing number of ova, the lining in your uterus continues to thicken until it reaches the point where it begins to fragment. At this point, irregular and often unpredictable bleeding occurs.[4]

They go on to caution that any abnormal bleeding should be checked by a doctor. There is usually nothing to worry about, but seeing a doctor is good preventive medicine: Increased bleeding can be a sign of cancer.

I have already recounted my frightening first experience with hemorrhaging. In all the books I have since read on menopause, there is very little said about more frequent bleeding except the consistent warning to check with your doctor. But I wanted the comfort of hearing other women tell me that they had experienced what I had. And what I didn't find in books, I found in interviews.

Many women had similar war stories of heavy bleeding. Perhaps women have been hesitant to talk about this symptom because it is so embarrassing. It is a situation that women feel they should be able to handle on their own. There is an attitude that, certainly by her mid-forties, a woman should be able to dress fastidiously, function with calm, and handle the logistics of her period without outside help. In the privacy of the group interviews, though, women readily expressed the discomfort and fear they felt about bleeding, and they agreed they would not have felt so overwhelmed if they had known that other women suffer the same thing.

Hemorrhaging is the most dramatic form of heavy bleeding. As with hot flashes, if you ask about hemorrhaging, you probably have not experienced it. It often means that you cannot be out in public and prevent bleeding through all protection onto your clothes. It usually requires medical attention because the bleeding can be heavy enough to cause anemia, a reduced amount of red cells in the blood. Alarming as all of this sounds, it is considered to be within the range of "normal" and things can be done to relieve the bleeding. The following stories give a sample of the help that is possible.

Debbie

Debbie is a manager in a large corporation. She is a petite blond who smiles a lot and is known for her encouraging personality. Her easygoing manner endears her to just about everyone and gives the impression that nothing much ruffles her feathers.

But Debbie now has an ongoing challenge to her ability to remain unruffled, with recurrent bouts of hemorrhaging. They began without warning when she was in her mid-forties. She started flooding at night. Then instances began to happen in the daytime. A D and C revealed no traces of cancer and temporarily cleared up the condition. But the hemorrhaging started up again after a few months. As Debbie recounted, she might be out to dinner with her husband and friends when the hemorrhaging would hit. After several trips to the ladies' room, she and her husband would have to leave so she could get home and off her feet. When that did not relieve the bleeding, she would head for the doctor's office again.

Debbie has had biopsies to rule out cancer but continues to live with the unexpected disruption of hemorrhaging. Her doctor put her on and off birth control pills for six months at a time to regulate her hormones and reduce the bleeding. This regimen has seemed to help.

Eileen

Eileen was in line for the submarine ride at Walt Disney World when she had her first hemorrhage.

"They [the staff at Disney World] took me to the clinic where they suggested I go to a doctor," she recounted. "I went back to my hotel room and saw a doctor later."

She rested the rest of the day and the bleeding slowed down. It was a frightening and embarrassing experience for her, but it was not abnormal. Eileen went to her doctor to verify that the bleeding was not from a cancerous condition, and needed no further treatment.

Linda

Linda was actually in the doctor's office when she started to hemorrhage. "At least I was in a place where I could get immediate help!" she said. She tried HRT but still had some bleeding problems, and finally had a hysterectomy to remedy the excessive bleeding.

Partnership with Your Doctor

The reason so many warnings are given about abnormal bleeding is because it can be a sign of endometrial cancer. Drs. Winnifred B. Cutler and Celso-Ramon Garcia define endometrial cancer this way:

Your endometrium is a gland that lines the central cavity of the uterus. The endometrium grows and thickens with each menstrual cycle, finally sloughing off during the menstrual flow. This tissue sometimes develops an overgrowth (a condition called endometrial hyperplasia), or, rarely, evolves into the more diseased state—the cancer.[5]

The idea of cancer is frightening, but for those who have verified the cause of their abnormal bleeding with their doctor, I have encouragement. Dr. Joe S. McIlhaney, Jr.'s book *1250 Health-Care Questions Women Ask* discusses irregular bleeding that does not persist month after month.

Most women who have abnormal bleeding worry about the cause being cancer, especially if it occurs when they are forty or over. It is important that a woman realize, however, that the cause of such bleeding is not usually cancer.

Remember, cancer is basically a "sore." As it grows it begins oozing a little fluid and then a little blood. Then, as time passes—perhaps weeks and months—that sore begins oozing more and more blood. This pattern of bleeding is quite different from the sporadic episodes of bleeding that almost all women occasionally have. The real key, though, is whether abnormal uterine bleeding is persisting.[6]

I had lain awake nights worrying that my irregular bleeding was a sign of cancer. It was a great relief to get the results of the D and C and the biopsy and find out this was not cancer. But I wish I had known, when I was going through those first frightening episodes, that abnormal bleeding is often a normal part of menopause.

Some women will not go for diagnostic testing because thay are afraid of the results. They just hope all is well and go on. But ignoring the possibility of cancer is gambling unnecessarily with your own body.

If you have abnormal bleeding, call your doctor and set up an appointment. Your doctor will probably perform an endometrial biopsy. This procedure is done in the office, usually without anesthesia. Your doctor will snip a tiny sampling of tissue from the lining of your uterus. That sampling is examined in a laboratory to determine if any of the cells are abnormal.

I have had an endometrial biopsy and found it untraumatic. There was an uncomfortable sensation for about ten seconds, and that was all. One woman interviewed, however, found it very painful and had resultant cramps. Discuss the possibility of anesthesia with your doctor if you are concerned that this procedure will be too painful.

If you have experienced hemorrhaging, your doctor may want to do a D and C. That procedure will not only allow for laboratory examination of cells but will usually clear up the abnormal bleeding. A D and C may also be done in the doctor's office with local anesthesia or in the hospital. Again, it depends on the individual. As I said earlier, I had a D and C in the doctor's office and experienced a minimum of discomfort. Other women I have talked with have been admitted to the hospital for D and Cs so that they can have general anesthesia.

The most important thing to do is to discuss in detail your personal options with your doctor. Don't be hard on yourself! If you are more comfortable being in the hospital under anesthesia, allow yourself to express that preference. Be sure that you have an honest, trusting relationship with your doctor, and do what you and your doctor feel is best for you. (See Chapter 7 for the importance of choosing a doctor during menopause.)

Suggestions for Survival

Sometimes, irregular bleeding persists even if you have a D and C. Reasons for this vary. You and your doctor can discuss your options, which may include a hysterectomy to end this particular symptom permanently. If you do not choose that route, here are other suggestions to make it through rough times:

- See your doctor.
- Have diagnostic testing done.
- In the meantime, carry tampons with you at all times.
- Continue to keep a calendar of your periods and note episodes of bleeding. This will help you and your doctor evaluate your symptoms.
- Talk to other women for encouragement.
- Try not to worry! As abnormal as this feels, for the most part it is normal for menopause.

CHAPTER 3

WHERE'S MY MIND AND WHERE'S MY WAIST?

N ow where was I? Oh yes, memory!

I began each one of my interview groups by asking the women how old they were. In one particular group, each woman wrote the information down on a piece of paper except for Elaine, who was fishing around in her purse.

I offered her paper and a pencil, but she said, "Oh, no, I'm looking for my pocket calculator."

"Your calculator?" I asked. The room became quiet.

"Yes," she said, still fumbling. "I can't remember how old I am. I can remember the year, but not how old I am now."

Elaine sensed all eyes turned on her and looked up from her bottomless purse. She saw traces of smiles appear and knew she had said something amusing.

"What?" she asked, smiling as well.

"Did you say you *forgot* your own age?" someone asked.

We all started to laugh. The familiar symptom of

memory loss had been demonstrated and the evening had just begun.

Memory Loss

Everybody experiences memory loss to one degree or another, but the kind associated with menopause is short-term memory loss. Dr. Wulf Utian explains it this way: "Recently, decreasing estrogen levels were linked to changes in short-term memory. The ability to remember immediate events, like the items on your shopping list, or to recall where you left your car keys or sunglasses can be attributed to declining estrogen levels."[1]

On a trip to California about a year ago, I had an exaggerated experience of this kind. I was staying with my older daughter in San Diego before going up to Pasadena to speak at a conference. The morning I was leaving San Diego I was the last one to leave Lisa's apartment. She and her husband had already gone to work and I was enjoying a leisurely morning.

I made several trips to load my car. After checking the apartment to be sure I hadn't left anything, I locked the apartment door and hid the key in a designated spot nearby. I slid into my rental car, put the key in the ignition, and then stopped.

Did I lock the door . . . or just hide the key? I asked myself.

I got out of the car and went back to the apartment. The door was locked. Back to the car.

I sat down, put the key in the ignition, and stopped again. *Had I locked the door?*

I got out of the car and went back to the apartment. The door was locked. Back to the car.

A third time the same doubt came over me. *Had I locked the door?*

This time I was able to overcome the urge to go back and check the door for the third time. *But not because I really remembered locking it.* I felt absolutely ridiculous. I pictured someone watching me from one of the apartment windows. They were probably on the phone right that moment calling the local hospital.

In one of the focus groups, Gail related how her memory loss had even impacted her enjoyment of reading. "I love to read, but I haven't in the last year because I can't concentrate." She couldn't remember enough to follow a plot from one night to the next.

Several other women described this loss of memory as "foggy" or "fuzzy brain." The sensation is one of clouded thinking; it takes a moment to call up information that used to be accessed quite easily.

"I was in a store the other day and the clerk asked me for my previous address. I couldn't remember the name of the street," Tammy said. Eventually she was able to pull the name up from her scrambled memory bank, but she described her brain as feeling fuzzy the whole time.

Interestingly enough, these women can function very well professionally. Remembering complex data doesn't seem to be as much of a problem as remembering what behavior they performed thirty seconds earlier or recalling a fact they have known for years.

Aids for an Ailing Memory

Some women report improved memory when they begin taking HRT. Others remember more accurately when they add vitamin B_1 to their diet.

Of course, the most obvious aid for compensating for memory loss is to write things down. I am a religious note taker. My memory became extremely overtaxed when my first husband was killed in a hot-air balloon accident over fourteen years ago. I had to close his business and raise two girls alone, and list-making became an integral part of my life.

My planner is jammed with all kinds of notes to myself. Disorganized as it looks, I can find what I need instantly. I am amused when I see planners that record only appointments, for mine has detailed lists of each day's activities. But my memory is pretty deficient! You may only need a simple list-taking procedure to compensate for the temporary memory deficiency that occurs during menopause.

Where Is My Waist?

I was sitting in the living room of a lovely home in California, listening to one woman after another express her frustration over the additional ten pounds (at least) she could not shed. Even as one woman was talking about her expanding waist, a loud "pop" interrupted her. Another woman's belt had burst open—a graphic visual aid of an annoying symptom of menopause.

I was blessed with a metabolism that allowed me to eat whatever I wanted until I hit forty. Nobody ever told me that metabolism changes as you enter the mid-life years. I kept on eating as usual, but I started to put on weight. Like so many other women, most of it seemed to be hanging around my waist.

Utian and Jacobowitz explain this metabolism change in *Managing Your Menopause*.

Beginning in your mid-thirties, and compounded by menopause, which usually begins in your early fifties, your food intake needs to be scaled back to accommodate your slower metabolism. Nature has rigged our basal metabolic rate (BMR) to slow down after the age of twenty-five, sliding between one-half and one percent per year. It happens gradually, so that it may be some time before you realize that you can't eat the way you once did. If you continue to consume the same amount of food that you have in the past, you will have difficulty keeping your figure.[2]

One woman commented on the irony of the situation, "Isn't it unfair? Most of us as kids were picky eaters. Then you grow up and you want to eat more and metabolism changes."

Weight gain is a physical symptom that isn't painful technically, but it can cause discomfort in a number of ways. Psychologically you don't feel good about yourself if you are dissatisfied with your looks. But even if you are not consumed with maintaining the weight you were at thirty, there is the challenge of getting used to how it feels responding to food intake differently. One woman said she couldn't get used to this new body. She had gained fourteen pounds during her forties and couldn't seem to lose it. She accepted her new look, but having been thin to begin with, she felt as if she no longer understood her own body.

Suggestions for Survival

Memory loss and weight gain are frustrating symptoms of menopause. In addition to a new planning notebook and a new belt, here are some things to think about when trying to live with these two changes.

- Remember—memory loss is normal and does not last forever.
- Be willing to use aids, like planning calendars and lists, without guilt. Many busy people with excellent memories use both.
- Try to reduce the level of stress in your life. Too much going on can result in memory overload.
- Be aware of the potential change in your body metabolism.
- Begin to train yourself to investigate low-fat eating.
- Go ahead and buy clothes that fit. Don't try to squeeze back into clothing that is too tight. You'll only feel guilty and depressed.
- Refer often to Chapter 8, which discusses diet and exercise.
- Uh . . . I forget the last one. But that's okay.

Emotional State of "Otherness"

"Take my hormones away, and I'll kill!" one otherwise rational woman said in the middle of a focus group. She had experienced such severe emotional distress during menopause that she was hospitalized at one point for psychiatric evaluation. HRT corrected this problem for her, and now she guards her hormones with vitriolic fervor.

Of course, she was kidding—kind of. Women who suffer from unstable emotions during menopause have a tough battle, given the perceptions associated with this symptom and the degree to which they may suffer.

Emotional distress is the descendant of the "hysterical female" syndrome of our grandmothers' day. It is the symptom that caused many women of menopausal age to be swept off to mental institutions and declared insane. The symptoms were seen as springing from the mind with no physiological basis. I have a friend in Florida whose mother committed suicide at the age of fifty-five (some forty years ago) because no one could help her out of her depression. She had been fine until her early fifties and then she suddenly changed. My friend attributes his mother's changed personality and subsequent suicide to undiagnosed menopause. He remembers his mother before she changed and does not believe she could have "just gone mad."

Fortunately, society's attitudes are changing. Emotional distress manifested as anxiety, depression, irritability, and crying spells has been studied and linked physiologically to the decrease of estrogen production.

Dr. Raymond G. Burnett, in his book *Menopause: All Your Questions Answered,* writes about this connection between decreased estrogen and emotional distress during the years prior to a woman's last period (the *perimenopausal* years).

> Many excellent studies now indicate that low levels of estrogen occurring in the perimenopausal years *do* have a definite physiological effect on important centers in the brain. In addition to hot flashes, the "withdrawal" from estrogen causes changes in the brain, which affect a woman's thought processes and lead to depression, anxiety, irritability, forgetfulness, insomnia, crying spells, lethargy, and fatigue. These are not symptoms of the woman who is ill-prepared for the menopause or the symptoms of a psychologically weak person. They are hormonally caused and have a physiological basis.[3]

Trapped in an Alien Body

I have always been a very emotional person. Just ask my daughters or my husband. "Mom cries at the playing of the national anthem at a football game," my daughters attest. "She even cries at the photos of dogs up for adoption in the newspaper. She's afraid they won't find a good home."

My emotions can certainly be effusive, but they are not the kind that lead to anxiety or depression. When I feel bad, I express myself openly. But the feelings of anger or frustration are over quickly, and lingering negative feelings are just not part of my personality.

Until a year ago.

Out of the blue, I experienced several attacks of feeling jangled, fragmented, anxious—totally unrelated to circumstances. Perhaps the best way to describe one of these attacks is to include the following journal entry.

Tuesday, November 9, 1993

I am undone. My nerves are jangled. I feel like someone took an egg beater—or a food processor—and surged through my insides. I don't feel sick, nauseated, physically unwell. But I AM NOT MYSELF. I am not even the "self" of me that is emotionally gushing. This is different. It is like being trapped in an alien body. What is happening? I have never felt this way in the past (prior to this last year). Even in times of great trauma in the past, I have been able to cope. I have been able to quiet my spirit before the Lord and go on. Now I am rattled, a mess.

Just this morning, I got out my at-home aerobic exercise step and started to exercise. I prayed that the endorphins would kick in quickly, and I would start to feel better. After thirty minutes of action-packed determination, I started to cry. Undaunted by the inconvenience of tears mingled with sweat, I kept on for another ten minutes. No good. Endorphins or not, I still felt like I just couldn't manage my body.

I pulled a chair into a sunny circle of the sunroom and sat down before the Lord. A heap. I was a heap. Sweating, crying, shaking—Lord, please help me. I knew that the Lord was with me. But no amount of spiritual fervor could take away the physical reality of dramatic changes going on inside my body. It was as if I had spigots inside me being turned on and off rapidly, releasing and cutting off some well-being fluid. I did not feel abandoned by the Lord, but I felt that a lot of things were going on that He intended to allow to continue. After a few minutes of crying out to Him, I called my doctor.

I explained how I felt to my doctor's nurse and that I had my daughter's wedding coming up in December and wanted to be semi-coherent for the big event. The nurse was wonderful—kind and reassuring. She promised me she would talk to my doctor and call back quickly. She did call back within twenty minutes and told me the doctor prescribed hormones for me to try until after the wedding and then we could reevaluate. Thank God. I am in such bad shape, I long for relief. Where is the old me? Where is the survivor? Deluged or dehydrated by the ebb and flow of internal controllers.

And so, I ask myself, If women who read this book want to know how these waves of "otherness" differ from emotional upsets in the past, what would I say? I would say that the main difference is that my methods for coping in difficult circumstances or during emotional upheaval—don't work. Even on the worst emotional roller-coaster rides, I have never felt unable to grasp onto truth in a way that calms the emotions. Now, I am aware of the truth but my body keeps me unwillingly on this scary ride. My faith and beliefs are intact, but the gears that slow down the roller coaster are disengaged. I pull the same levers, but the ride only speeds up.

This is about coping. I have often been called a survivor, so this inability to cope with feelings makes me mad. I want to rise above the circumstances. I want to will my body to behave. I want to trust that the Lord will give me that amazing grace to which I have become so accustomed. It is not about faith. I have talked to many Christian women who have felt guilty because their faith could not get them through this passage of life without medical help. Faith is not measured by accepting assistance for stress versus gutting it out on your own. Help comes in many forms. For women in hormonal stress, one of the ways help comes is through hormone replacement therapy. It is not the only way, but it is a way that is as acceptable to the faith-filled believer as it is for anyone else.

Hysterectomies and Emotions

More than one-third of the women I interviewed (31 out of 105) had undergone hysterectomies. A hysterectomy may or may not include removal of the ovaries. If it does, the production of estrogen in the body is stopped abruptly. Those women interviewed who had their ovaries removed and who were not put on hormones immediately told of often severe emotional ups and downs. The sudden total lack of estrogen in their bodies caused this symptom.

Naomi said, "I woke from the surgery and felt out of

control. I was crying uncontrollably. It was like watching myself go nuts. This young girl was pushing me from one room to another in a wheelchair and she kept bumping me into things. I started screaming and crying."

For Naomi, the waves of emotional irrationality continued. She asked her doctor about them and he said it was all in her mind. He told her that her body had healed, but her mind had not. His insensitive manner propelled Naomi into another frenzy. It also propelled her to seek the advice of another doctor. Her new doctor put her on HRT, and within a few weeks Naomi was back to normal.

Emotions That Are Difficult to Define

Even the most emotional women interviewed expressed that menopausal emotions are different from what they usually experience.

"I just don't feel myself," Ann said. "I feel emotionally out of control. I feel fragmented."

On an intellectual level, reason prevails. Most women in the middle of emotional distress know that they are feeling out of the ordinary. They are aware of what is happening. But the intellect seems to be held captive by emotions. It is a frightening loss of control. Even trying to explain this distressing symptom of menopause, a woman can fall short of adequate communication.

That Elusive Sense of Well-being

"I don't have real discernible mood swings," Lynn said when talking about emotional distress, "but I have noticed a general sense of free-floating anxiety. In the last few years, I just seem to be a little anxious, a little apprehensive, like something bad is going to happen."

Lynn is not alone. Many women express the same

general sense of anxiety. They may not feel out of control, but a once-routine sense of well-being seems to be missing.

Personally, in my thirties I felt as if I had stopped flitting around in life and had reached some peaceful plateau. Now that flitting feeling is back. It's not all the time and not always severe. But there are times of uneasiness that resemble periods during my high school days when the future was uncertain.

There are times in our lives when the future *is* uncertain. We will look later at life circumstances that do have an impact at mid-life. But this elusive sense of well-being is less connected to the circumstances of objective reality than it is to free-floating, upredictable angst.

Suggestions for Survival

Women going through menopause are *not* crazy. Even though women in earlier times were often misdiagnosed and carried off to institutions, today there is no need to fear such extreme reactions. Today, there is help.

- Many women, after consulting with a doctor, are put on HRT with great success. This will be discussed in full in the next section.
- Many other women find vitamin supplements helpful, including vitamins B_1, B_3, B_{12}, C, and calcium.
- Evaluate the level of stress in your life and try to alleviate problem areas.
- Make sure you have some quiet time away from the hustle and bustle of everyday life, even if it means excusing yourself during the height of an activity.
- Ask the Lord for a sense of peace to help you get through the day.
- Talk with other women for encouragement and hope.

• Find a doctor who will work with you on solving this challenge in ways that are affirming to you.

Fatigue

"I used to be a night person," Elaine said, "and now I start to nod off around nine o'clock. My husband can be sitting reading or watching television, and I fall asleep sitting up."

Elaine occasionally has night sweats that interrupt her sleep. Fatigue is a predictable result. Other women in her focus group experienced increased fatigue and blamed it on changes in their metabolism. Endless energy or that second burst of steam that used to kick in after dinner is a thing of the past. They feel lethargic since the onset of menopause, and a slower metabolism has caused weight gain and decreased energy.

"I feel weighted down," Mary said. "I eat the same as I used to but have gained weight and, as a result, feel more tired."

Some women found relief by reducing their calorie intake. Others simply tried to rest during the day if they felt tired. Exercise also proved a great boost to the system and increased the level of energy.

Dizziness

A few women who suffer from hot flashes experience dizziness at the beginning of a hot flash. Others have bouts with dizziness and no accompanying hot flashes. But generally the spells last only a few seconds and are not debilitating.

If you feel dizzy, sit down and wait for the dizziness to pass. Get up slowly and take your time moving around. Usually, the sensation is corrected with a few minutes of rest.

If dizziness persists or is severe, see a doctor. He will check you to rule out causes other than menopause. Some women also experience dizziness as a side effect of taking HRT. Doctors can alter the treatment to eliminate the dizziness.

Loss of Libido

Some women experience changes in their sexual desires. Unlike the supposed oversexed, hysterical female of history, the women I interviewed sometimes lost interest in sex during menopause. They attributed their change in desire to fatigue, emotional ups and downs, hot flashes, and vaginal dryness.

This symptom was one that women in the focus groups rarely talked about openly. Rather, they came to me privately to admit that they had a decreased interest in sex.

One attractive, vivacious woman told me that she hated to admit her lack of interest openly because it was such a contradiction to how she had enjoyed her sexual relationship with her husband all their married life. Because of a strong family history of breast cancer she could not take HRT. No other treatment, like vitamins or diet changes, seemed to help. She and her husband were trying to talk honestly with each other, as she underscored that this symptom was not a personal rejection of her husband. Fortunately he believed her and was willing to work with her on ways to restore intimacy. At this writing, great passion hasn't returned. But their loving relationship allows for sexual expression that is less frequent than before but still meaningful.

Some women believed that relieving symptoms like stress and fatigue helped to restore their interest in sex. Overall lifestyle also seemed to be important. Women agreed that reducing stress, spending time away with their husbands, and taking care of themselves so that they felt attractive helped rekindle old flames of desire that had been extinguished with the multitude of changes during menopause.

A Comprehensive List

The following list includes the symptoms that have been discussed, as well as a few dozen more. They are categorized into three types: autonomic (involuntary symptoms), physical and metabolic changes, and psychogenic changes.

The word *psychogenic* means "originating in the mind or in mental conflict." This does not mean that these symptoms are some kind of mental illness. As cited earlier, there is evidence that many of these symptoms are a result of decreasing estrogen in the body. They have a physiological (characteristic of or promoting normal, healthy functioning) basis with a psychological manifestation.

This particular list is taken from *Menopause and the Years Ahead,* by Mary Beard and Lindsay Curtis.

1. Autonomic (involuntary symptoms)
   hot flushes   palpitations of the heart
   hot flashes   night sweats
   cold chills   increased perspiration
   angina pectoris
     (chest pains)

2. Physical and metabolic changes
   menstrual changes
       changes in cycle (shorten or lengthen)
       changes in flow amount (increase or decrease)
   breast-size decrease (atrophy)
   skin thinning and wrinkling (atrophy)

vaginal atrophy (dryness, burning, itching)
   discharge and occasional bleeding
   dyspareunia (painful intercourse)
   contracting and scarring of tissues
   shortening and narrowing
vaginal relaxation with prolapsing (falling out of
   position)
increased facial, chest, and abdominal hair
bladder dysfunction
   frequency of urination
   dysuria (burning or stinging sensation when
      passing urine)
   increased bladder infection
   bladder infection symptoms without infection
osteoporosis
increased muscular weakness
degeneration of bone joints
increased cardiovascular disease (heart attacks
   and strokes)
3. Psychogenic

apathy	frigidity
apprehension	headaches
decline in libido	insomnia
depression	irritability
fatigue	mood changes
forgetfulness	
formication (feeling like ants under the skin)[4]	

After reading this list of symptoms, you may feel ready to pack your bags and head for the hills. Do you want to be around people if you are sprouting hair on your face, breaking bones with every step, forgetting your name, and scratching furiously at imaginary ants under your skin?

But remember the teeming masses of women ahead of us who are a testimony to survival! The next two sections look at what treatments are available and how to decide which ones are right for you.

CHAPTER 4

....

EXPLAINING
THE CONTROVERSY

....

Menopause is a normal process of life. All women who live long enough experience it. Some of them don't feel badly at all. So why talk about treatment as if every woman has to make a decision about it?

There are two reasons why women need to understand the treatment controversy and how to make decisions about it.

1. Distressing symptoms of menopause can be greatly relieved. It is important to know what treatment is available and what controversy currently exists with regard to treatment in order to make wise choices.
2. Even if women do not experience menopausal symptoms, they may be subject to osteoporosis and heart disease. Treatment for menopausal symptoms also includes beneficial treatment in the prevention of these two diseases.

Normal does not mean that a condition does not need attention. Menopause is normal, but it needs appropriate care. Every woman should educate herself on the treatment controversy and consider how to best apply numerous choices for treatment to herself. She may choose not to make any changes in her personal health regimen, but at least she will be making a choice based on current, relevant information.

Does Every Woman Need Treatment?

Before researching this book, I had no idea there was such a heated controversy over the treatment of menopausal symptoms. In the last few years, however, this controversy has been the topic of numerous books, articles, and seminars. Much of the information women get is one-sided, and many women make decisions without seeing the whole picture.

Passions run deep beneath the scientific-sounding proclamations of how women should respond to menopause. The controversy is so emotionally charged that it leaves many women limp with confusion as to who is right.

There are, basically, two sides in this debate: the opinion of medical establishment and the opinion of those who favor nonmedical methods of treatment. In between there are numerous blends of the two that seek benefits from the best of both worlds. Many doctors do incorporate nonmedical methods, like exercise, in their treatments for menopause. Fewer nonmedical advocates endorse taking HRT. And that is the crucial issue in the debate: whether to take HRT or not.

Medical advocates appeal to the promise of enhanced quality of life without distressing symptoms and the added protection against osteoporosis and heart disease. They persuasively paint a picture of necessary medical intervention in most women's lives from menopause until death.

Proponents of a nonmedical approach to menopause proclaim the virtues of living without potent chemicals coursing through a woman's body for half her life. They paint an equally persuasive picture of menopause as a normal stage of life which requires no medical intervention.

This section will not advocate a particular position but outline the controversy and present the differing views (including risks and benefits of each). Included are the choices some women have made, my own personal process of evaluating treatment, ways to make intelligent decisions, and a challenge to be proactive in your own decision making.

The discussion can be simplified by looking at four general areas: hormonal changes that cause symptoms, medical treatment, nonmedical treatment, and blended treatment.

Hormonal Changes That Cause Symptoms

The symptoms of menopause are caused by the cessation of the production of the hormones *estrogen* and *progesterone*.

A woman is born with as many eggs as she will ever have. These eggs are found in the ovaries, and each egg is surrounded by a follicle (sac with fluid). It is this follicle that produces the hormones estrogen and progesterone. As a woman gets older and loses eggs (encased in the follicles that produce estrogen and progesterone) through menstruation or atrophy (decreasing in size), less estrogen is released in her body.

Progesterone, simply stated, is the hormone that prepares the lining of the uterus for pregnancy. If pregnancy does not occur, the lining of the uterus sloughs off and menstruation is the result.

When the ovaries have depleted their supply of eggs, menstruation stops, hormone production of estrogen and progesterone stop, and menopause occurs.

Estrogen and progesterone affect many parts of the body and, when they cease to be produced, the whole body changes. Hence, the presence of menopausal symptoms as well as the cessation of periods.

A *hysterectomy* is the surgical removal of the uterus and ovaries. This operation results in what is called *surgical menopause*. No matter what age a woman is at the time of a hysterectomy, she may suddenly experience menopausal symptoms, such as hot flashes, mood swings, and forgetfulness, because she no longer has ovaries to produce estrogen and progesterone.

Medical Treatment

Hormone replacement therapy is the medical community's answer to the negative impact of menopausal symptoms (see Chapter 5 for a complete discussion of the benefits of HRT). During the early years of HRT, estrogen was given alone. The lining of the uterus still thickened, but it did not slough off because of the absence of progesterone. This condition was believed to cause a rise in incidents of uterine cancer. To help prevent possibilities of uterine cancer, the treatment was changed to include progesterone with estrogen, thus producing the desired shedding of the lining of the uterus. Therefore, women on HRT that includes progesterone continue to experience monthly bleeding. They are not menstruating but still experience the bleeding as a result of this needed elimination of the lining of the uterus.

HRT is given in a number of ways: pills, shots, implants, vaginal creams, patches, and creams. There are also a number of possible combinations of hormones that a woman may be given, but most of them consist of a dosage of estrogen combined with a dosage of *progestin* (the name of the progesterone replacement product.)

Examples of possible treatment dosages are found in Utian and Jacobowitz's *Managing Your Menopause:*

- You take estrogen tablets on days one to twenty-five of the month and add progestin for approximately twelve days (days fourteen to twenty-five).
- You use the estrogen patch, changing it twice weekly for twenty-five days and take oral progestin on days fourteen to twenty-five.
- You take one of the other estrogens and progestins in equivalent doses and cycle twenty-one days on and seven days off therapy.[1]

Ways to administer hormones are as individualized as the dosages. Doctors seek to prescribe the smallest dose possible to relieve the individual's symptoms.

The popularity of this treatment among obstetricians and gynecologists is documented in the article, "The Raging Hormone Debate." Writer Amanda Spake reports, "A whopping 75 to 95 percent of ob-gyns surveyed said they would prescribe hormones—either estrogen alone or in combination with progestin—to most of their recently menopausal patients."[2]

Nonmedical Treatment

The proponents of nonmedical treatments prescribe the use of vitamin supplements, diet, exercise, herbal therapy, and other miscellaneous treatments. (This is not to say that the medical community does not recommend proper diet and exercise, but those components are not included in their primary therapy.) And the strictly nonmedical approach does not recommend HRT.

Advocates of the nonmedical approach think there is an overmedicalization of menopause. They believe that since menopause is a natural process of life it can often be effectively treated without medical methods.

Ann Louise Gittleman, nutritionist and author, believes that poor nutrition and negative lifestyle habits have been bypassed as possible contributors to menopausal symptoms. She explains her premise in her book *Super Nutrition for Menopause*.

> This last conclusion [poor nutrition and negative lifestyle habits] is really the foundation of this book. My research into the whys and wherefores of this life passage began pointing to unbalanced body chemistry as a potent underlying cause of menopausal woes. While about 75 percent of all women experience distressing symptoms purportedly connected to declining estrogen and progesterone, the remaining 25 percent do not suffer any adverse effects. Why? The answer, and perhaps the key solution to menopause, is found in the little-known fact that the reduced amount of estrogen and progesterone from the ovaries is naturally compensated for by hormones produced elsewhere in the body, primarily the adrenal glands and body fat, nature's back-up system. This hidden piece of vital information is a nutritional clue as to why some women suffer through menopause and others don't. When our bodies are overstressed, our adrenals can become exhausted and this natural back-up system fails, leaving us unprotected, and making menopause far more difficult than Mother Nature intended it to be.[3]

Gittleman goes on to emphasize the damaging effects of dietary and lifestyle choices prior to mid-life that negatively impact health at the time of menopause. She encourages her readers to consider making diet and lifestyle changes that will improve health, even after years of poor choices.

Lear's magazine had a short comment on this issue of lifestyle choices that supports Gittleman's opinion.

A recent report in the *Journal of the American Medical Association* suggests that the top causes of death "are all rooted in behavioral choices," such as smoking, drinking, a sedentary lifestyle, and a high-fat diet. Tobacco, the authors say, claims approximately 400,000 lives annually; poor nutrition and lack of exercise, 300,000; and alcohol, 100,000. Which means there's a lot you can do to save your own life.[4]

The nemesis for the nonmedical advocates is lack of verifiable results. They do not have the research behind them that the medical community has. That issue—funding for research—is also a part of the controversy. Some proponents of nonmedical treatment believe that funding for research is minimal because big business (like pharmaceutical companies) is not behind them.

The vitamin industry advertises claims of relief from menopausal symptoms but has recently come under attack for these and other undocumented claims. In 1990, Congress stepped in with new controls on the vitamin industry's labeling claims:

The Nutrition Labeling and Education Act requires health claims to have "significant scientific agreement among experts based on the totality of publicly available evidence." The FDA has the right to preapprove all claims for accuracy.[5]

This means that menopausal women shopping in health food stores for vitamins to relieve their symptoms may soon find manufacturers' claims to be more restrained.

The biggest plus on the side of the natural therapies is that they do not usually cause negative side effects. And they certainly are not linked with anything as serious as cancer. Women who take this approach base it on this added safeguard and on effectiveness of relieving symptoms.

A Blended Approach

Some women—and researchers—have chosen to take a middle road between the medical and nonmedical approaches. Among the most famous of these is Dr. Wulf H. Utian. Dr. Utian is a world-renowned obstetrician-gynecologist with a Ph.D. in reproductive endocrinology, who established the world's first menopause clinic in South Africa. He is currently the Executive Director and founding President of the North American Menopause Society in Cleveland, Ohio. He also developed the Utian Menopause Management Program which blends HRT and some nonmedical components in treatment of menopausal women.

The eight essential tools of the Utian Program are:

1. You, yourself.
2. A physician whom you trust and respect.
3. Hormone treatment may work for you.
4. The right diet.

5. Exercise that makes you look and feel great.
6. Total body care.
7. Wearing clothes that suit you.
8. Finding menopause clinics and support groups.[6]

Most doctors would agree with Utian on the necessity of right diet and exercise, but the emphasis of the medical community is on HRT. Utian, while he agrees with his own profession as to the benefits of HRT, also puts an emphasis on nonmedical methods as well.

....

CHAPTER 5

HISTORY OF HORMONE REPLACEMENT THERAPY (HRT)

....

*B*y now you may be thinking, "Enough, already. I don't care if relief is spelled H–R–T or V–I–T–A–M–I–N–S." This is taking too much mental energy, and your energy is lagging with every turn of the page. It would be so easy if there were only one preferred, undisputed opinion and a woman could say, "Amen, that's the route for me."

The problem is that one of the most prescribed treatments, hormone replacement therapy, carries with it a potentially life-threatening risk. Women who listen to only one side of the treatment controversy may wind up making a dangerous choice.

The history of HRT is an illustration of what has happened to some women who did listen to just one side. Women who responded to dramatic, untested claims of estrogen as a miracle cure, jumped on the bandwagon thinking they were headed for utopia. They took estrogen for relief of menopausal symptoms, but some of them ended up with uterine cancer.

That problem was corrected and all seemed well until the question was raised of a possible connection between HRT and breast cancer.

Reviewing the history of this debate can help you make more informed personal decisions, based on all the factors in this complicated issue.

The First Appearance of Estrogen

In the 1920s, scientists linked the fluctuation of body hormones with women's menstrual cycles. Since the hormone estrogen ceased to be produced in women's bodies after menopause, the medical community looked for a way to replace that estrogen and, thereby, relieve menopausal symptoms. By the 1930s, estrogen was being prescribed for relief of those symptoms.

Estrogen replacement therapy, or ERT, was the official term for estrogen treatment. It was prescribed from the 1930s to the 1960s on a limited basis but skyrocketed to success in 1965 with the publication of the book *Feminine Forever*, by Robert A. Wilson. Wilson made elaborate claims as to the benefits of ERT which did prove to relieve menopausal symptoms greatly.

Wilson's sexist language, declaring that women needed to take estrogen to remain beguilingly alluring to their husbands and keep their flaming passions alive, would not win him favor with many women of the 1990s. But in the 1960s he found an enraptured audience.

Feminine Forever

Feminine Forever put ERT at the top of the list of wonder cures for women. Wilson's strong language inferred that any woman who did not take estrogen was foolish. He used the word *castration* to describe the cessation of estrogen production in the body.

Estrogen therapy was not to change a woman, Dr. Wilson insisted.

> On the contrary: *it keeps her from changing*. Therapy does not alter the natural hormone balance. Rather, it *restores* the total hormone pattern to the normal, premenopausal level. Whether this is interfering with nature or restoring nature is a moot point. The results speak for themselves.
>
> So much for the medical side of the argument. If the question is to be examined on philosophic grounds, I rest my case on the simple contention that castration is a bad thing and that every woman has the right—indeed, the duty—to counteract the chemical castration that befalls her during the middle years. Estrogen therapy is a proven, effective means of restoring the normal balance of her bodily and psychic functions throughout her prolonged life. It is nothing less than the method by which a woman can remain feminine forever.[1]

The book includes chapters entitled "Menopause—the Loss of Womanhood and the Loss of Good Health" and "Plain Talk About Sex." In these chapters, he paints a totally dismal picture of the menopausal woman and appeals to the men of his day with a frank discussion of enhanced sexual relations with women who take estrogen. He discusses a "Femininity Index" which analyzes the types of vaginal cells taken by a pap smear:

> Three types of cells are visible on the slide: superficial, intermediate, and parabasal cells. The cytologist in his laboratory makes a careful count of all three cell types. This count answers one of the most crucial questions

that ever confront a woman. It tells whether her body is
still feminine, or whether it is gradually turning neuter.[2]

Wilson goes on to explain to husbands that if their
wife is below par on the Femininity Index, estrogen will
correct the problem and bring her index up to full femininity.

Apparently some of Wilson's medical cohorts did
not approve of his strong argument for hormone replacement based on restoring women to peak sexual
performance. To strengthen his case, Wilson enlisted
endorsement from men in the ministry.

> Most clerics, however, have been sympathetic to my
> work. Knowing through their counseling work the
> depth of domestic misery often brought on by un-
> treated menopause—ministers, priests, and rabbis are
> often more receptive to the idea of hormone therapy
> than the more traditional-minded members of my own
> profession.[3]

Feminine Forever is mentioned in most discussions
about the history of estrogen therapy. It is considered
the benchmark publication that had menopausal
women in the 1960s beating a path to their doctor's offices to get prescriptions for the wonder cure for van-
ishing femininity.

Trouble in Paradise

Wilson's claims that ERT worked may have proved
satisfactory, but his claims of ERT being safe came
crashing down in the late 1970s with the reported rise
of endometrial cancer among women taking estrogen.
Endometrial cancer is cancer of the lining of the uterine
cavity, commonly called *uterine cancer*.

As Amanda Spake recounts in her article, "The Raging Hormone Debate":

> A decade later, after thousands of women were using the drugs, the bad news started to trickle in: Women on estrogen had eight times the risk of uterine cancer and might have upped their risk of breast cancer as well. Suddenly, the glory days of estrogen appeared to be over.[4]

The New England Journal of Medicine published a shocking report on February 1, 1979, entitled, "Replacement Estrogens and Endometrial Cancer." It was the definitive medical data used to substantiate the link between endometrial cancer and estrogen. The results were summarized as follows:

> The present study confirms that long-term replacement estrogen treatment is strongly associated with endometrial cancer. Furthermore, in these data discontinuation of estrogen intake is associated with a striking decrease in risk of endometrial cancer within six months. Whereas the annual risk in non users is about one per thousand, the annual risk among all current users is very high—of the order of 20 per thousand. Among long-term users, the risk is even higher.[5]

Correcting the Dominant Problem

Since estrogen replacement therapy was meant to mimic a woman's natural cycle, doctors considered introducing progesterone into this therapy, the hormone that causes the sloughing off of the lining of the uterus. Women who were taking estrogen alone had replaced the estrogen in their bodies, but not the progesterone.

They were not experiencing the necessary sloughing off of the lining of the uterus, which at times was leading to endometrial hyperplasia. Hyperplasia advances in stages which can eventually lead to cancer.

Drs. Cutler and Garcia explain this change in hormone treatment in *Menopause: A Guide for Women and Those Who Love Them:*

> The development of estrogen replacement therapy began with the use of estrogen alone (that is, unopposed). It is only recently that progesterone has been routinely added to estrogen therapy in an attempt to mimic the natural cyclical pattern of the fertile years. This addition protects the endometrium from developing cancer to which it would otherwise be at risk by the unopposed estrogen therapy. Once progesterone was added to estrogen therapy, the name of the process began to change—from estrogen replacement therapy (ERT) to hormone replacement therapy (HRT).[6]

Breast Cancer and HRT: History in the Making

The addition of progesterone to estrogen seems to have solved one problem that occurred in the history of HRT. But then the question was raised: Is HRT related to the development of breast cancer?

The opinions of doctors vary on the subject of breast cancer risk while taking HRT. One strong advocate of the safety of taking HRT without fear of breast cancer is Dr. Lila Nachtigall, Associate Professor of Obstetrics and Gynecology at New York University School of Medicine and Director of the Women's Wellness Center at NYU Medical Center. In her book *Estrogen, A Complete Guide to Reversing the Effects of Menopause Using Hormone Replacement Therapy,* this highly credentialed woman boldly tells women that estrogen is safe: "Estrogen replacement is absolutely safe when it is used correctly in the new medically proven way (in low doses, combined with progesterone, prescribed individually, and monitored regularly)."[7]

While other doctors agree with Nachtigall, they are not as quick to use terms like "absolutely safe when used correctly." Drs. Cutler and Garcia, mentioned earlier, stress that the decision with regard to risk is up to the individual.

> In any case, you should know that there is a risk whenever you take a medication. No one knows for sure what the effects will be for a specific person. Every experience in life carries with it some risk. . . . From the abundance of rigorously designed studies, the increased risks of properly dosed hormones appear to be low, provided that you are not in the "should not take hormones" category.[8]

Utian and Jacobowitz voice what the medical community does agree on—careful monitoring of women on HRT (Chapter 6 provides a list to help determine if you are in a high-risk category).

> In all instances, the strong recommendation is for an annual mammogram while on HRT and a semiannual breast examination by a physician, in addition to breast self-examination. As an added plus, the development of any breast problems that are unrelated to HRT will be diagnosed earlier as well.[9]

Gretchen Henkel is a writer who has been covering medical and health topics for over fifteen years. She quotes several doctors in her book *Making the Estrogen*

Decision, who express strong skepticism as to the merits of HRT.

> The question of potential breast cancer risk with long-term HRT is "very difficult," says Dr. Karen Blanchard. "There are very good studies that show there is no increased risk of breast cancer, and there are studies that show that there *is* increased risk. Well, we live in a society where one out of nine women get breast cancer. *Every* woman is at increased risk of breast cancer in our society. However, I don't think the entire picture has been developed, and we'll probably need another generation before that can be answered in an intelligent way."
>
> "What about breast cancer?" asks Dr. Lewis Kuller. "Well, that's the big IF. We don't really completely understand the possible interrelationships. In the past, most women who got estrogen therapy were given it because they were symptomatic during the post menopausal period. And, those women, by definition, are deficient in estrogen, so they are probably at lower risk of cancer, if estrogens are related to cancer.
>
> "Unfortunately," continues Kuller, "the NIH [National Institute of Health], which should have done these trials 15 years ago, is just now in the process of embarking on such trials."[10]

Paula Dranov, a writer of health and medical material, summarizes the research in her book *Estrogen: Is It Right for You?*

> Earlier studies of the breast cancer-estrogen connection were much more reassuring. Most showed no increased risk at all, and some actually suggested that estrogen protects women: they found less cancer among the estrogen users than among the comparison groups.

Today, most researchers give more credence to the newer studies and agree that estrogen replacement does increase a woman's risk of breast cancer and that the risk may be higher still when a woman takes progestin as well as estrogen.[11]

The following warning is from a printed insert that accompanies a video promoting Premarin (conjugated estrogen tablets). The video, *Premarin: What Every Woman Should Know About Estrogen,* is produced by Ayerst Laboratories (the makers of Premarin) and is used by doctors to give to menopausal women as they decide whether to take HRT or not.

This warning is written under the subhead "Dangers of Estrogens."

> *Cancer of the breast.* The majority of studies have shown no association with the usual doses used for estrogen replacement therapy and breast cancer. Some studies have suggested a possible increased incidence of breast cancer in those women taking estrogens for prolonged periods of time and especially if higher doses are used. Regular breast examinations by a health professional and self-examination are recommended for women receiving estrogen therapy, as they are for all women.[12]

Tamoxifen: Friend or Foe?

There is another hormone involved in the breast cancer controversy. Paula Dranov outlines the possibilities for tamoxifen.

> Tamoxifen, a synthetic hormone used to prevent recurrence among women with estrogen-dependent breast cancer, is being studied as a means of preventing breast

cancer in healthy women. In 1992 the National Cancer Institute launched a five-year study in which 16,000 women will be given either tamoxifen or a placebo. If tamoxifen proves as effective a preventive measure as some researchers suspect it will, all post menopausal women may be advised to take it for the rest of their lives![13]

Dranov goes on to discuss the potential negative side effects of tamoxifen, including severe menopausal symptoms, liver disease, and endometrial cancer.

Confusing? You bet. HRT is strongly endorsed by many, endorsed with reservation by some, and regarded with greater caution by others. In addition to the potential benefits of relief from menopausal symptoms, there are other benefits of HRT to consider.

Other Potential Benefits of HRT

Despite its rocky history, HRT provides benefits that improve health and quality of life for thousands of women. The two most noted are prevention of osteoporosis and prevention of heart disease.

Osteoporosis is a serious disease. It is a condition of weakened or brittle bones that can break easily, seen most in women after menopause. One woman said that her mother had had her backbone replaced when she was in her thirties with the backbone of a sheep. Another woman was still in her forties but had been tested for bone density and told she already had serious bone deterioration.

The New England Journal of Medicine came out with a report on October 14, 1993 entitled, "The Effect of Postmenopausal Estrogen Therapy on Bone Density in Elderly Women." The conclusion of the report stated:

For long-term preservation of bone mineral density,
women should take estrogen for at least seven years
after menopause. Even this duration of therapy may
have little residual effect on bone density among
women 75 years of age and older, who have the highest
risk factor.[14]

There is also a great deal of talk in the medical community about the positive effects of HRT in the prevention of heart disease or coronary artery disease (CAD).

Dr. Marianne J. Legato in her book *The Female Heart*
says:

> What has proven to be of most interest to internists and
> cardiologists, however, is that a handful of studies also
> confirm that women on HRT have a 30 percent to 50
> percent reduction in the development of CAD compared with menopausal women not taking any replacement therapy.[15]

It is reported that heart disease kills more women
than cancer. Legato says, "40,000 women die of breast
cancer each year; 250,000 will die of a heart attack."[16]

So many medical professionals see the benefit of
heart protection to outweigh the possible risk of cancer.

Where We Stand in History

New research and new objections continue to appear
on the scene. One book that was published in Australia
in 1991, has now made it to America: *The Menopause
Industry: How the Medical Establishment Exploits Women*,
by Sandra Coney.

Coney has been writing on women's issues for many
years with a focus on women's health. She takes exception, among other things, to the widespread prescribing

of HRT as a preventative medication without appropriate publicity given to the fact that these hormones are potent drugs.

> There is no discussion of the wisdom or ethics of medicating huge numbers of asymptomatic well women with powerful drugs. This is not recommended for any other drug or for the prevention of any other condition. Even with heart disease in men, the major killer for the over-47-year-olds, anti-hypertensive drugs are only recommended for those with clear indications. The switch from HRT as a treatment, to HRT as preventive therapy has occurred without debate or justification. It is a shift of the profoundest significance, yet has gone unremarked and undiscussed.[17]

And so we stand at a crossroads. What will be proven about HRT remains to be seen. Tests are being conducted now that will reveal to our daughters' generation who is right: the people who strongly endorse HRT or the ones who express great caution in taking it.

We have to decide without the advantage of conclusive results. That uncertainty makes the decision-making process pretty important.

CHAPTER 6

BEGIN WHERE
YOU ARE NOW
....

*I*f you are in the very early stages of menopause, you may not need to decide on any specific treatment yet. Early stages would mean that you still have fairly regular periods and experience only mild symptoms. Maybe you skip a period every few months and have had hot flashes once or twice.

You are fortunate because time is on your side in this decision-making process. You can apply these suggestions for making decisions and not be pressed by overwhelming symptoms that demand immediate attention.

If you are already experiencing distressing symptoms, you may want to read this section quickly and get started right away in the decision-making process to determine the best treatment for you.

If you are already involved in treatment for menopausal symptoms, this section may be helpful in evaluating your choices. In any event, the result will be increased confidence in making the best choices for you.

It's Time for an Attitude Check

There are several ways to choose a course of action without really choosing.

- Ride with whatever happens and hope for the best.
- Take your doctor's suggestion without further investigation.
- Do what your best friend is doing.
- Do what your mother did—if you even know what she did.

Many women opt for one of these nonaction approaches. Just a few weeks ago I ran into an old friend I had not seen for a few years. She asked what I was doing, which led to a discussion about menopause. I asked her if she took hormones. She said she didn't and had never spoken to anyone about the subject. After her last child was born, over twenty years ago, she stopped going to a doctor.

"If anything is wrong," she smiled, "I don't want to know about it."

She has chosen to ride with whatever happens and hope for the best. That may work fine for her as long as she has no adverse health conditions such as cancer, osteoporosis, or heart disease. But if she does develop health problems, she will have missed the opportunity to prevent major illness.

Check your own attitude. Are you a passive bystander when it comes to decisions about your health? Do you rely on your doctor or other people to make decisions for you?

The first step in navigating the middle years of life is to realize that you can enhance the process of aging, including menopause, by being actively involved in decisions about your own health. You don't have to do what your friends do, or what your doctor says, or what your mother did. You can become informed and choose what is best for you.

New information flows off the presses weekly about women's health. Studies are in progress today that will alter what treatments are recommended tomorrow.

This process of making decisions about your health will be ongoing and not always simple, but it can be fun. Try not to think of it as another chore to accomplish, but an enhancement, not an interruption. It can happen in the context of your everyday life. It can involve other women. You will be encouraged and have a greater sense of control by active participation in making the important decisions about your own well-being.

Surveying the Data

There are twenty-six books about menopause on the floor next to me as I write this book. I have read all or parts of all of them. They range from strictly medical books to the spiritual musings of middle-aged women.

They are written from a number of different perspectives with conflicting suggestions about treatment and attitudes. Some are humorous and others are very serious. Some are medical books that give detailed explanations of the physiological process of menopause. Others focus on in-depth nutritional regimens to follow.

Because there is not a consensus on the subject of menopause, it is important for a woman to read a wide range of books with a critical eye. There are statements in some books that are contradicted in other books, so it is crucial to evaluate the author's perspective and temper conclusions with an understanding of the bias.

For instance, if a medical doctor has written a book, he or she will most likely be in favor of HRT. Knowing that, you can read the book understanding that the benefits of HRT will be highlighted more than the potential risks. On the other hand, a book by a nutritionist will probably be against taking HRT. You can read that book to learn about the benefits of nonmedical methods of treatment, well aware of the bias on HRT.

More and more newspapers and magazines are carrying articles on menopause. Develop the habit of scanning publications for this topic. It has been said that *knowledge is power*. Learning more about menopause will only aid your decision-making process.

Evaluating Your Own Risk Factors

Remember the journal entry about my hysterical phone call to my doctor requesting hormone pills?

Well, I only took those frantically ordered pills for eleven days. I got dizzy, and then I got scared. In my panic to take care of the immediate crisis, I had disregarded a critical component of good medical procedure: looking at risk factors.

I do not know my family medical history because I am adopted. I don't know that the dizziness was caused by the pills, but it stopped when I stopped taking them. Family medical history plays a key role in deciding what kind of treatment you will take. You will see in the lists in this section that family history appears in four of the five lists. That incident set me on a course of study as to why women may or may not be candidates for HRT.

Risk Factors in Taking HRT

In *Managing Your Menopause,* Dr. Utian says that he will not prescribe HRT for women with any of the following:

• Known or suspected breast or uterine cancer or any other estrogen-dependent tumor (a tumor in which estrogen will stimulate growth)

- Strong family history of estrogen-dependent cancers
- Abnormal and unexplained genital bleeding
- Dubin-Johnson syndrome (chronic jaundice—a liver problem) or chronic liver disease
- Acute liver disease[1]

The list goes on to list other conditions that do not rule out use of HRT, but require careful evaluation:

- Uterine fibroids
- Endometriosis
- Hyperlipidemia or hypercholesterolemia (conditions of abnormally high concentrations of fat or cholesterol in the blood)
- Severe varicose veins
- Diabetes mellitus
- Porphyria (metabolic disturbance that can cause acute abdominal or nervous problem, or photosensitivity of the skin or sores on its surface)
- Severe hypertension
- Previous or present thromboembolism, or severe thrombophlebitis[2]

Risk Factors in Developing Breast Cancer

Even though there is disagreement about the relationship between HRT and breast cancer, there does seem to be agreement on one important issue. Dr. Marianne Legato writes about estrogen-dependent cancer in her book *The Female Heart:*

> It is also important to point out that the growth of some types of breast cancer is enhanced by estrogen; if a woman has a previously undetected and estrogen-sensitive tumor of the breast, and begins to take hormone

therapy, her cancer will grow faster than if she is not taking estrogen.[3]

Dr. Lila Nachtigall agrees:

It is absolutely essential to know whether an existing breast malignancy is or isn't dependent on estrogen for its growth.

HRT must never be given to anyone with an existing estrogen-dependent cancer because, although it was not responsible for initiating it, it can make this kind of cancer grow more rapidly.[4]

What if you have never had breast cancer detected? It makes sense to evaluate your risk of developing it before deciding on treatment.

Dr. Linda Ojeda in *Menopause Without Medicine* lists the following risk factors for breast cancer:

- Heredity: Risk is greater for those whose mothers, aunts, or sisters have had it.
- Age: Older women are more at risk.
- Country of birth: North American and Northern European women have increased risk.
- Socioeconomic class: Higher-income families have increased risk.
- Race and religion: White women have higher incidence than black women and Jewish women have twice the risk of non-Jewish women.
- Marital status: Never-married women have higher risk than those who have been married.
- Menarche: Early menarche (under 12 years) increases risk.
- Menopause: Late menopause (over 55 years) increases risk.

- Childbearing experience: Having had no children or having a first child after age 30 increases risk.
- Weight: Being overweight increases risk.
- Shape: Weight distributed in upper body and stomach increases risk.
- Diet: Poor diet increases risk.[5]

Risk Factors in Developing Uterine Cancer

The other cancer risk linked to HRT is that of uterine cancer. This risk has been dramatically reduced with the introduction of progesterone into the hormone regimen. But some researchers still believe it is a potential risk. The FDA still requires manufacturers of estrogen medication to include warnings in their packaging that estrogen has been reported to increase the risk of endometrial cancer.

Drs. Beard and Curtis describe women more likely to develop cancer of the endometrium (I have presented their information in list form):

- Women whose ovaries secrete too much estrogen
- Women who do not ovulate or those who have what we call *dysfunctional* (abnormal or irregular) uterine bleeding
- Women who have had no children
- Women who have high blood pressure
- Women who have diabetes
- Women who have obesity[6]

Risk Factors in Developing Heart Disease

So far, we have been evaluating reasons to be cautious about taking HRT. But there may be advantages of taking HRT to consider in addition to relief of symptoms of menopause.

As mentioned in Chapter 5, there is evidence that estrogen helps to protect against heart disease. Consider (without the intervention of estrogen) the following risks of heart disease, as listed by Utian and Jacobowitz.

General Risk Factors: (apply to men and women)
1. High blood cholesterol
2. Hypertension
3. Diabetes mellitus
4. Obesity
5. Poor Diet
6. Cigarette smoking
7. Physical inactivity
8. Stress
9. Family history of heart disease

Women-Only Risk Factors:
1. Menopause before age forty-five
2. Surgical menopause
3. Low estrogen level
4. Use of oral contraceptives[7]

Risk Factors in Developing Osteoporosis

Estrogen has also proven to be helpful in preventing osteoporosis. Ojeda lists the following as risks for this crippling disease.

- Has any member of your family had bone disease?
- Are you thin and small-boned?
- Are you fair-skinned?
- Were your ovaries removed before age 45?
- Are you childless?
- Have you been confined to bed for an extended time?
- Are you a diabetic or hypoglycemic?

- Are you lactose intolerant?
- Do you have an underactive thyroid gland?
- Do you have diabetes or kidney or liver disease?
- Are you sedentary?
- Do you avoid dairy products?
- Do you smoke cigarettes?
- Have you been involved in prolonged dieting or fasting?[8]

Using These Lists Effectively

These lists can be confusing. How can they help you make a decision and not frustrate further your decision-making process? Follow these steps to see more clearly what risks you have:

1. Go back over the lists and put a check next to any risk that applies to you.
2. Count the check marks from the first three lists—risk factors in taking HRT, risk factors in developing breast cancer, risk factors in developing uterine cancer.
3. Count how many risk factors you have in the last two lists—risk factors in developing heart disease, risk factors in developing osteoporosis.
4. Look at the first three lists to see if any factors indicate high risk for taking HRT.
5. Look at the last two lists to see if any factors indicate high risk for heart disease or osteoporosis.
6. List the risks side by side with the benefits.
7. Use this information with other suggestions in this chapter to help you make a decision.

Let me show you my personal results as an example.

List #1—Risk in taking HRT	1
List #2—Risk of breast cancer	5
List #3—Risk of uterine cancer	1
List #4—Risk of heart disease	1
List #5—Risk for osteoporosis	1

In the lists where I had a risk factor of 1, it was due to my lack of family history. So, it could just as easily be a 0. I ranked it as 1 because of my own personal concern. If I felt no concern, I would rank that risk as 0.

My conclusion, then, is that my primary area of concern is in risk of breast cancer. Notice that the list of breast cancer risks includes older North American women. These indicators give many of us an automatic 2 risk number. I still have an additional 3 risk factors for breast cancer.

In evaluating the data, then, the biggest issue for me in deciding whether to take HRT or not is how I view the risk of breast cancer. As well, my own personal conclusion is that the argument for taking HRT to protect against heart disease and osteoporosis in me (given my health) is a weak one. However, my confidence is tempered by the reality that we never know for sure how long our bodies will hold up.

Try evaluating the lists for yourself, and make some conclusions based on your own personal risk factors.

CHAPTER 7

INVESTIGATE OTHER RESOURCES

*A*re you a clipper?

A clipper is a person who cuts articles out of newspapers and magazines and saves them for current and future reference. All you need to clip successfully are a pair of scissors and some file folders.

Information is pouring off the presses on the subject of menopause. If you don't organize some way to keep it, it will be of little value to you. This book can be a helpful guide through the maze, but you will also probably want to find a little corner of your home—a drawer, a portion of a file cabinet, a box under the bed—and start compiling the information that is meaningful to you. You can set your files up in any way that works for you. Some possible file labels might be: hormones, nonmedical approaches, diet, exercise, personal stories, new research discoveries, "my feelings." It may be helpful to include book titles, doctors' or clinic names, friends who have been helpful. Remember, your memory may start to lag! Writing notes about good ideas or even stashing away journal entries will help you evaluate your changes in your body and your thoughts.

The previous chapter gave a survey of the current scientific data available. But there are three other sources of information to be tapped into: the experiences of other women, specialized medical resources, and specialized nonmedical resources.

Listen to Other Women

I have so much fun talking to women about their personal experiences during menopause! Even after I finished with the wonderful, warm focus groups organized for this book, I have continued to talk to many women. I am always greatly encouraged after a conversation with another wanderer on this winding road through mid-life.

Part of the encouragement comes from women being so open to share and so eager to listen. It is certainly true that no one understands the perils and pitfalls of menopause like another woman experiencing the same thing.

Of course, there are some women who don't feel they are experiencing anything difficult and resent being asked to talk about aging. They do not want to talk about being old, or older, or over-the-hill, or members of the menopause category. They deny missing any beats in the rhythm of their lives and wonder what all the fuss is about. That's okay. This is individual stuff. If they are blessed to be among the few women who never have an unpleasant menopause symptom, then they probably will have little to share with those of us who have plenty to talk about. (However, given the treatment controversy discussed earlier, all women would probably benefit from talking with other women about menopause.)

So if you are looking for other women to talk to, you may encounter a few who don't appreciate the subject matter. But I don't think you will run into many. Even women who have not started the process of menopause yet are usually very interested in discussing what lies ahead for them.

Forty-nine percent of the 105 women I interviewed are taking HRT. But many of those women were not thoroughly comfortable with their decision. They wondered about how long they should continue the treatment, uncertain that they want to remain on any drug for the rest of their lives. Most of them had varying degrees of fears about cancer. For these women, even reassurances from their doctors fell short of convincing them to endorse unconditionally this method of treatment.

A smaller number of women were totally enthusiastic about HRT. Most of these women had suffered such severe menopausal symptoms that the risk factors were less important than the quality of life they had finally regained while on HRT. The chaos experienced without HRT was too devastating.

Among the 32 percent of women who decided not to take HRT, the same ambivalence existed. Some had opted not to take it because their symptoms were not completely disrupting the quality of their lives. But they wondered if they were adding to their risk of heart disease or osteoporosis. Others were passionately against taking HRT because they felt it was unproven, unsafe, or unnatural treatment.

The 19 percent who had not decided are still listening.

Here are some stories of women in all three categories. You may recognize your own thoughts, questions, and emotions as you hear what they are experiencing.

Ruth

Ruth is fifty-seven years old and has been on HRT for eight years. She has a pap smear every year and an endometrial biopsy every other year because of previous spotting between periods. Ten years ago she had a breast lump biopsy that was benign. At the focus group, she talked about how she felt HRT was wonderful because she feels fine, her skin is in good shape, she has no emotional ups and downs, and she is guarding against osteoporosis.

Jill

Jill has suffered from repeated hemorrhaging. She has been tested and, thankfully, has no signs of cancer. Her doctor had been suggesting HRT for some time before Jill agreed to try it. Her mother has had breast cancer, but the doctor was not worried because her mother was in her seventies when the cancer appeared. Jill went on HRT for a few months, then off for a few months, then on again in an attempt to regulate the bleeding. HRT did help her problem with hemorrhaging, but her worry over possible cancer continued. She finally decided to stay off HRT despite her doctor's recommendation that she keep taking hormones. For Jill, the apprehension about cancer was greater than the benefit of the HRT. Since she went off HRT, the hemorrhaging has not returned. Jill is hopeful that whatever HRT she did take corrected the hemorrhaging and that she is past the worst of the symptoms.

Barbara

Barbara is one of those rare women who just doesn't seem to worry. She is in her mid-fifties and has been on

HRT for three years. She is a personal advocate for HRT but agrees that it is not for everyone. Her biggest concern about her health as she ages is that of osteoporosis. Barbara also feels that a lot of women put undue stress on their marriages if they do nothing about their emotional symptoms during menopause. She has had none of these symptoms either before taking HRT or since she has been on it. Barbara takes estrogen as a preventive measure and intends to stay on it indefinitely.

Beverly

"I am not on HRT and don't intend to ever be on it," says Beverly, a vivacious, outgoing woman in her mid-fifties.

Beverly sports a beautiful year-round tan, due partially to living in Florida and due partially to her natural olive complexion. A very attractive woman, she told of her doctor's initial reason for recommending HRT to her.

"Your skin would look better if you took HRT," he said during a routine visit.

Beverly was frank about her response to his comment. "I remember thinking to myself, *I don't think my skin looks so bad!* I didn't tell him how little I appreciated his comment. I just decided to continue with my skin as it is and forget the HRT."

Mariann

Mariann, fifty-seven, is an enthusiast of nonmedical treatment. In her late forties and early fifties, she had severe bouts with mood swings but opted to treat them with vitamins instead of HRT.

"Everything would get out of proportion," she recounted. "My voice level would rise and I'd get looks from my family. I would get jangled and antsy and my family knew not to disagree with me. I started taking vitamins and stopped drinking coffee after breakfast."

Mariann went on to say that the vitamins did help her. Because she never seriously considered HRT, she determined to make it through rough symptoms no matter what.

Gladys

Gladys was the first one in her group to speak up in favor of HRT. She had had a hysterectomy at age forty-four. Before the hysterectomy she never had any menopausal symptoms. After the surgery, she was automatically put on hormones. Gladys said she felt better than she had in years.

"I didn't know that I felt bad before the surgery. But afterwards, I just felt so much better on HRT," she said enthusiastically.

She has been on HRT for five years and thinks it is the best thing that has ever happened to her.

Sue

In another group, Sue began the discussion by admitting that she is a self-professed advocate of an all-natural approach, but she is taking HRT.

"I was learning a new job at work. I would sit at my computer and cry and pray no one would see me. I would cry when doing dishes. Then the sleeplessness started and the migraines. My doctors said I should be on hormones. I didn't want to but decided to try. Once on them, I really leveled off. Until my last son graduates, I will not give them up."

Sue said she still favors a natural approach but her

symptoms were interfering with her life to such a degree that she had to do something that would really work for her.

Laura

Laura had a hysterectomy at age forty-five after several years of heavy, painful periods. After the hysterectomy, she went on HRT at the advice of her doctor.

"I was on hormones for three and a half years, and then my doctor died. I took myself off and have been off for fifteen years. I don't have any problem, so I don't take any medication."

Laura talked about how she changed from automatically taking a doctor's advice to thinking for herself. She admitted that it took the death of the doctor she had seen for many years to get her to think about what she really wanted to do. But before she went to another doctor she decided, regardless of his advice, she didn't want to take HRT anymore.

Pam

"I guess I am one of the few people who has negative side effects to hormones," Pam told the ten women in her group.

She was the only one in that group who had tried HRT and couldn't continue to take it because of those adverse reactions.

"I went to the doctor and she put me on [HRT] and it made me very angry. It kind of changed my personality. I was slipping into depression and had 'foggy' brain. A friend of mine went to a nutritionist. So I went too and came home with a ton of stuff. I am now symptom-free."

Pam said she had not been a supporter of vitamins

before trying them for menopausal symptoms, but after she couldn't take HRT and still suffered severe menopausal symptoms, she thought it was worth trying. It has worked for her. She takes various kinds of vitamins and recommended that anyone who wanted to try this approach should talk directly with a nutritionist.

Elizabeth

Elizabeth is one of the women who struggles with her decision about treatment. She has been on and off HRT for five years. She has a fear of cancer and doesn't like the prospect of long-term drug use, but her symptoms make life difficult without HRT.

"I was on it for a while and took myself off because of the fear of cancer. I found that I felt much better on it, so I went back on. I am concerned about what the long-range problems might be, but for now, I am doing well."

Jackie

Jackie is fifty-eight years old and started taking HRT because of heart disease in her family. Her doctor recommended it as a preventive measure.

"I would not have gone on hormones except for the family history of heart problems," she said. "I went off them for a few months and my sleep was so disturbed— I would startle awake fifteen to twenty times a night. So I went back on hormones."

She is still on HRT but wishes she were not. She feels ambivalent all the time about whether she is doing what is best for her health.

Linda

Linda is a quiet and reserved school teacher. She is one of those people who never loses her temper. But

Linda told a story about altered personality when she went off HRT for a short time.

"I had taken myself off HRT just to see how I would feel. I had been on it for over five years and just thought I'd like to know how I felt without it. After about two weeks, I was at a teacher's meeting one afternoon and got really agitated with one of the men teachers. He was debating an issue for the sake of debating and was holding the whole group up. I was sitting next to him getting madder and madder. He wouldn't shut up. Finally, I jumped up and grabbed him around the neck and shook him. He looked so shocked. Then I sat down and didn't apologize for what I did. Later, I thought to myself, *You better get back on hormones right away!*"

All of these stories are unique. Each woman has evaluated the seriousness of her symptoms, her personal health risk factors, her fears, and what treatment would best fit her personal needs. These stories confirm that there is no one right answer to the question of how to treat menopausal symptoms.

Investigate Specialized Medical Resources

Some of my friends do not go to doctors. They have discounted the medical community completely since they entered the age of menopause. Even if you choose a nonmedical approach to treatment of menopausal symptoms, seeing a medical doctor is probably wise for routine diagnostic tests.

After advocating such a strong position for making personal decisions, why am I saying unequivocally, do this? Because I don't think it is wise to ignore the use of preventative diagnosis. It is possible to find a doctor only for check-ups or preventative testing. Do be open and explain your skepticism of the medical community.

But also be willing to listen. If you have a distressing diagnosis—such as cancer detected by a mammogram—
you are still open to choosing the treatment you want to
take advantage of.

The good news is that there are increasing types of
medical practitioners to consider. One that is especially
helpful for menopausal women is the nurse practitioner. A *nurse practitioner* is a nurse who has advanced
training and is able to do more than a registered nurse
but less than a doctor. Exactly what they can do is reg-
ulated by the individual state in which they practice.

Nurse practitioners work under the umbrella of a
physician. They perform mid-level services and allow
doctors to focus more on surgery and problem areas.
For instance, in many states nurse practitioners can administer pap smears and prescribe medication. If they
find a problem with a pap smear, the patient can then
be referred to the doctor.

There are also nurse practitioners who specialize in
women's health. They allow more time per appointment
than most doctors so they can discuss with each patient
particular concerns—which may or may not be related
to the reason for the visit. A pap smear, for example,
only takes about three minutes, which is so brief a
woman has no time to talk with the doctor. A nurse
practitioner allows extra time to answer questions and
has the time to "just talk" about menopause and the
merits of different treatment. They are also able to give
advice and relate experientially at the same time. A
female gynecologist may or may not provide the same
atmosphere of competence, understanding, and avail-
ability for you. If your regular doctor is a man, seeing a
female nurse practitioner as well may enhance that existing relationship and not pose a threat to the profes-

sional relationship. The best way to find any professional is by personal referral, but if you hit a dead end that way, you may want to try your phone book.

I grew up around a lot of doctors. My father seemed to know a number of men in medicine, and they were his personal friends as well as doctors who treated my family. I trusted these men. They were dear to me, and I accepted their word on medical issues as unchallengeable truth. Most of my life I have had positive relationships with men in medicine, but that is not always the case for women.

The quality of relationship with a doctor who is going to advise you during menopause is crucial. It is unnerving to be treated condescendingly by a doctor when you are talking about real symptoms. It is equally frustrating to be dismissed as "too young" or "simply imagining things."

There are many wonderful doctors to be found, but sadly, some still treat women as if the mental illness myths of the 1900s were current reality. If you find yourself in an uncomfortable relationship with your doctor, look around. Ask your friends. You have no reason to stay with a doctor who will not be helpful to you during this time of life. Your doctor is a primary resource of information and individualized attention. It is worth taking the time to find a man or a woman you can trust and to whom you can talk openly.

Menopause Clinics

Another medical resource that is becoming more prevalent in the United States are specialized divisions of hospitals or specialized clinics associated with various hospitals. According to the North American Menopause Society there is no comprehensive list of such clinics at this time, but there are some eight or nine centers in the United States. Your local hospital may be able to refer you to one nearest your home. The closest one to me is The Women's Mid-life Health Center at Swedish Medical Center in Denver, Colorado. The center's coordinator, Helen Ricles, graciously allowed me to attend the center's day-long clinic as an observer. It proved to be a wonderful experience that I wholeheartedly endorse.

I was not a patient, so I do not have a personal financial statement to illustrate specific costs. The Women's Mid-life Health Center's "One Day Health Assessment" requires a nonrefundable processing fee of $25.00 (rates as of December 1993), which is applied to a $75.00 center fee. Other fees are determined by the testing used—pap smear, mammogram, blood work, and more. Each patient consults with a staff person at the clinic prior to her day's assessment. At that time, the relevant tests are determined and she can contact her insurance carrier to see what is covered. The cost depends on testing and on insurance coverage.

I was to arrive at the clinic at seven A.M. I felt ashamed of myself when I arrived at the clinic suite with coffee in hand. Two women, Doris and Linda, were patients that day, and since they were having blood tests that morning they had not been allowed to eat or drink anything. I gulped my last swallow of coffee guiltily.

Helen Ricles, the two women, and I settled comfortably in a little conference room that was to be our meeting center for the day. Helen explained the day's format—lab work for them, back to the conference room for instruction, lunch, more instruction, afternoon appointments for them with the doctor who would give them the results of their morning tests, and final consultation with Helen.

One of the big advantages of this day-long program is finding out test results the same day. The agony of wondering what the mammogram or pap smear will show is over by the time you go home. While mammograms are often read right away, under normal doctor's office conditions pap smear results can take up to two weeks to find out.

While Doris and Linda went for their tests, I viewed a video on symptoms of menopause. They rejoined me shortly, and after coffee (this time for all of us) the instruction began. We studied charts that detailed exactly what happens to a woman's hormones during menopause—very technical but very interesting. Helen answered many questions that came up, and we were amazed at how much about our own bodies we did not know.

Another session was on breast health. The clinic had sample "breasts" made of a mushy kind of material with simulated cancerous lumps in them. It was fascinating. I have had benign breast lumps before and have always wondered how the doctor can tell by touching them that they are probably not malignant. Handling these sample "breasts" answered my question.

We talked a lot about benign breast condition because it is so common: One out of three women experience it (myself included). It is frightening because it appears as a lump in the breast, the same way cancer can appear. These benign cysts often begin to show up around the same time other menopausal symptoms do, because of hormonal changes. I thought how helpful it would be if all doctors had sample breasts so that women would know what they are feeling for when doing self-exams.

Other sessions included a complete explanation of HRT and personal nutrition assessments for Doris and Linda. Each woman had her consultation with the doctor and final discussion with Helen. At the end of the day, recommendations were given regarding individual treatment.

The atmosphere was warm, personal, and focused. The health personnel in menopausal clinics are working every day with menopausal women. They have access to the latest medical data and incorporate nutrition and other lifestyle components into their program. Women who can spend a whole day with professionals and talk about their individual treatment plans have access to so much more than was available just a few years ago. If there is a menopausal clinic near your home and if your insurance will help cover the costs, it is well worth investigating.

There are also increasing numbers of seminars popping up across the country targeting the mid-life woman. The easiest way to find out about any in your area is to call your local hospital. Ask for their women's division—many hospitals now have separate women's sections—for information on upcoming seminars, or watch for announcements in your local newspaper.

Nonmedical resources are also available through health food stores and nutritionists. One way to find out what your city offers is to check the yellow pages (health food stores, vitamins, nutritionists) and the newspaper.

Repeat the Process

Since menopause does cover a number of years in your life, you keep changing and so does the research regarding treatment. Even when physical symptoms wane, life circumstances, relationships, and your own thinking need shoring up. So don't think of this decision-making process as a once-and-for-all event. It is ongoing.

Here is a summary of the process we have covered in this section.

- Begin with an attitude check. Are you content with being passive in decisions about your own treatment? Think about being more proactive.
- Read a wide range of material from differing viewpoints.
- Evaluate your own risk factors.
- Organize and file away pertinent information, helpful insights, or journal entries.
- Listen to other women.
- Research specialized medical resources.
- Research specialized nonmedical resources.

Pay Attention to Your Intuition

Remember my journal entry with the frantic call for hormones? I felt dizzy for a number of days before I listened to my intuition that the hormones could be causing the problem. We are all, to one degree or another, making educated guesses based on contradictory information. But intuition can play a very important role in your decision making, for you are the only one who can sense what is happening in your own body.

I remember anticipating glowing results from taking hormones. A friend of mine had experienced exactly the same symptoms I had—she still had her period but was having anxiety attacks and forgetfulness. She went on hormones and felt better almost instantly. I expected the same thing to happen to me. When it didn't, I was surprised. Why wasn't my body responding the same ways her body was? I don't know, but it wasn't. I had to pay attention to my own body and realize that I didn't feel good on the hormones. That may change in the future; for now, it isn't good for me to be on hormones.

No matter how fast or slowly you make decisions, it is okay to change your mind. You can't rely on someone else's experience to predict how you will respond, and you can't predict what your own experience will be prior to a specific treatment. So pay attention to your intuition.

Involve God in the Decision-making Process

God is not on vacation while a woman moves through this often stormy time of life.

In the midst of a specific decision-making process, a woman especially needs to stay closely connected to God the Father, Son, and Holy Spirit. I am not a proponent of the legalistic performing of religious activities, but I do know that my life is fuller, richer, and more peaceful when I come into the presence of the Lord daily. I ask Him for guidance in *all* matters—pills, doctors, tests, discernment in the midst of conflicting information. He has not given me a vision of a prescription tablet with one answer written on it, but He has given me a sense of peace as I daily try to make wise decisions.

Section 5 includes ways to improve spiritual well-being. Putting some of the suggestions in that section into practice will also help your ability to sense how God is leading you in the specific area of decision making.

CHAPTER 8

I DON'T WANT TO READ ANOTHER WORD ABOUT DIET AND EXERCISE!

I know what you're thinking. You want to skip this chapter because you already know what will be written about diet and exercise, and it will not be fun. I agree. Oh, that we could just eat what we want and lie around like we like, and all would be well.

I like sweets, but I *love* fats. One of my favorite treats is to put butter (real butter, not any low-fat variety of almost-butter) on chocolate cake. Yes, I said *cake*. My father taught me this little-known delicacy and let me tell you, it is wonderful! And of course, corn on the cob is a traditionally excellent vehicle for more butter. When I was growing up we lived about two hours south of New York City. My family would go to Coney Island in the summer to spend a day riding the Steeplechase and roller coaster and pause between rides for a drenched-in-a-vat-of-butter ear of corn.

My mother often declined this indulgence because she was not blessed with the galloping metabolism my father and I enjoyed. He made up for her reticence. He was the consummate food lover. I remember many nights when my father, unable to go to bed without a full stomach, would wake me up to join him for a bacon, lettuce, and tomato sandwich. We could munch away and go right to sleep. No nightmares or sleepless nights because of overworked digestive systems for us!

What I don't remember is one word of caution when I was growing up about too much fat, and I remember only a few words about rationing sweets. The words from experts would not have mattered to my father anyway. He loved food and relished every mouthful. And since he didn't like to dine alone, I was his cohort in high-fat consumption.

We have both been spared, so far, the ravishing results of high-calorie intake. Most people are not so blessed. (I am well aware of God's gracious blessing of a high metabolism.) I have great empathy for people who could never get away with indulging in such a state of decadence.

For all of her life, my mother gained weight simply by being within ten miles of food. She could almost starve herself and still weigh more at the end of the day than she did that morning. This seems decidedly unfair.

Menopausal Metabolism

By mid-life, however, the scales begin to strike a balance. Those of us who have escaped having weight problems join the masses in the battle of the bulge. I am sadly aware that my metabolic processes no longer burn up those fat calories like a furnace but rather at the pace of dying embers.

So whether you have always been on the diet roller coaster or not, the need to face the diet monster is a must. I promise not to bore you with suggested meal plans or rules about counting calories, all of which you have been reading for years. But do hear the warning you already know: Being overweight, especially as you age, can severely damage your health.

There are volumes written about how to lose weight. You can purchase calorie-counting guides in editions the size of encyclopedias or ones that will fit in your purse. Nothing I can say here will change your way of eating if you are not convinced it will be worth the Herculean struggle to attempt to change. Overcoming unhealthy eating habits is not easy, but any safe effort is worth pursuing. You really will feel better, physically and emotionally.

A Healthy Attitude Shift

An earlier chapter mentioned the notorious ten pounds that usually arrive with menopause. I have still not been able to shed them. I tried my usual crash diets to no avail, and finally accepted that I will never again weigh what I weighed most of my adult life.

This is not all bad news. Because I had been relatively thin most of my life, I could afford to gain ten pounds and not be overweight. The acceptance of my current weight has more to do with a change in attitude about what is attractive. After a lifetime of aiming at *thin*, I am finally letting go of the idea that the lingerie models are the norm for all of womanhood (not that I ever did have a shape anything like those sculpted forms).

Being thin is not necessarily equivalent to being healthy. We can be so consumed with weighing what our teenage daughters weigh that we can deny our bodies healthy nutrition in pursuit of a wispy look. My current weight is well within healthy guidelines for a woman my age and frame. It is not thin, but it is not fat.

If you have struggled with being overweight, maybe you need an attitude shift for a different reason than I did. Most women interviewed who needed to lose weight admitted that they had wanted to lose weight in order to look better. But mid-life brings into focus the issue of health. The lists in Chapter 6 for evaluating risks for breast cancer, uterine cancer, and heart disease all include obesity as a risk factor.

Whatever you weigh as you enter menopause, *the important fact to realize is that your metabolism has changed.* If you continue to eat what you always have, you will gain weight. If you cut down, you will lose or maintain weight.

To maintain or reduce your weight at mid-life Utian and Jacobowitz's *Managing Your Menopause* recommends:

Average/Active Woman—2,000 calorie lifestyle.
Average/Occasional Woman—1,600 calorie lifestyle.
Overweight/Nonexerciser—1,000 calorie diet style.[1]

Wonderful Little Books

Since I really had no comprehension of how many calories are in any given food, I did buy one of the pocket-sized calorie-counting books. It also includes a column for how many of the calories are in fat. If you check out one of these handy little books, it will explain the percentage of fat calories a day that are suggested to maintain your desired weight.

Wait a minute! you may be saying. *You weren't going to tell us to count calories.*

I'm not. But low-fat diets are the optimum way to eat. Studies continue to determine the link between high-fat diets and disease. By familiarizing yourself with which foods are high in fat and which ones are not, you can evaluate the pattern of what you eat and how much fat content it has.

I carried my calorie-counter book with me for only about three weeks. It amazed me to see how some foods I grab on the run—especially fast foods—are extremely high in fat. So I changed some habits. If I knew I would not be able to stop in a restaurant for a balanced lunch, I would take an apple and a bag of pretzels with me. Eating on the run is not the ideal way to eat, but it is a fact of life for many of us. Simply substituting something from home can cut hundreds of calories and fat out of the daily intake.

After a while, you will know which of your favorite foods are high or low in fat. Cantaloupe is very low in fat and potato chips are very high, so I now choose the cantaloupe as a snack instead of the high-fat potato chips. Mayonnaise is much higher in fat than mustard, so I put mustard on sandwiches instead of mayonnaise.

The change is much more difficult with high-fat foods that have no satisfying substitute. Personally, I feel deprived when I eat a piece of bread and don't load it up with real butter. There is just nothing as good! But I am learning to put *less* butter on the bread—a start.

Chocolate Once a Week and Fruit Every Day

I had to teach myself to eat fruit. Fruit doesn't contain fat, so it doesn't satisfy me the way the buttered chocolate cake does.

The conversion to fruit is happening, though slowly. To help myself learn to reach automatically for fruit, I try to make it very accessible. I keep a bowl of washed grapes out on the kitchen counter during the day. Then, when I walk through the kitchen, with an urge to eat something, I grab a few grapes. If they were in the refrigerator, I don't think I would go looking for them. (What would be more automatic is to go to the cupboard where the potato chips are, as I have for years, and grab a handful.)

I love fresh squeezed orange juice. We lived in Florida for about twelve years and regularly bought this delicacy by the gallon in grocery stores at a reasonable cost. I remember the first time (and only time) I saw fresh squeezed orange juice in a store in Colorado. I excitedly picked up a gallon and went to the checkout line. When the clerk got to the orange juice, she looked up and said, "Do you realize that this costs ten dollars?"

"Ten dollars for a gallon of juice!" I was in shock.

I took it out of my order and decided to stay with the frozen concentrate. A few years ago, though, I bought a juicer. Not one of the new fancy ones, just an electric dome-shaped device. But it does the trick. I buy economy bags of oranges that are meant to be used for juice and keep the oranges out on the counter in a bowl. Seeing them, like seeing the grapes, reminds me of a healthy snack that I might otherwise miss.

I am convinced that I will go to heaven with my desire for chocolate still active. To keep me from becoming obsessed with a not-so-healthy treat, I allow myself to have a little once a week. If I know that I am not banned from the pleasures of chocolate for eternity, I can usually last until the weekend to indulge my sweet tooth.

The Honest Struggle

I will be very honest and admit that I have not reached the point where I do not long for my favorite high-fat foods. Oh, some days are better than others. I can go for longer periods of time without having chocolate cake with butter. But the old days of carefree eating are fond memories, and I do yearn for them at times.

The value of changed eating habits is what keeps me hanging in with repeated attempts at better, healthier food choices. I really do feel better when I maintain my weight at the new adjusted level. When I go over, I feel sluggish and uncomfortable. My self-esteem drops because I don't like how I feel, as well as not liking how I look.

If you are seriously overweight or underweight, do consult a doctor. Aging increases stress on your body that is greatly impacted by diet, and it can cost you your life.

I don't go to Coney Island anymore. The days of midnight bacon, lettuce, and tomato sandwiches are over. But I feel good. I can change how I eat. And I get better. Just this morning I had raisin toast—without the butter.

What Works for You

How many times have you read the come-on: *A Diet and Exercise Plan You Can Stick To?* Even more than with dieting, few women have found a way to stay with consistent exercise.

The ones who do manage to work out regularly agree that exercise, like eating well, is an ongoing discipline. Of the women in the focus groups, several of them walked a few miles every other day, some played tennis, and some went to aerobic classes. Very few worked out with weights at all.

I never considered working out with weights until I began research on menopause. Almost every book on the subject recommends weight-bearing exercise to help prevent osteoporosis. Proponents of both medical and nonmedical menopause treatments stress the danger of deteriorating bones and urge women to do these exercises. I decided to check it out.

I have been a member of a health club for years. A typical routine is to make a New Year's resolution to work out three times a week. I do this religiously for two weeks, then I drop down to twice a week. Then guilt takes over and I throw out the whole plan.

Last year I made a decision again. Lethargic, depressed about weight gain, and upset with myself for failing so miserably every time I tried to establish a workout program, I dusted off my health club card and ventured back to the gym. My club, like most of them, offers a free demonstration on the machines with a trainer.

Oh yeah, I thought. *A trainer. A body-perfect, pumped up, muscle-bound . . . guy.*

I had a long conversation with myself about the foolishness of not doing something because of my pride. *You are a mound of flab. You need to work your body into better shape or the mound will only continue to grow. You need to admit that you are almost fifty and will never again look like you are twenty-five. You need to admit that muscle-bound trainer doesn't care how you look. Call. Make the appointment.*

I called. I made the appointment. I cried.

How did I get to feeling so badly about myself? I had put off for years the decision to discipline myself to exercise. I could not call those years back, but I could begin to improve for the remaining years, which, after all, might be considerable.

On the appointed day, at the appointed time, I appeared in the lobby of the health club, dressed in my workout gear and ready to go. The receptionist told me to take a seat and the trainer, Marie, would be right out.

Marie? I thought. *A woman!*

She would undoubtedly be decked out in a drop-dead aerobic outfit that highlighted the difference in her body and mine. Then the unthinkable happened. The receptionist told a weight-lifter-type guy to join me. He and I were to have a joint session with Marie.

I wanted to run. A middle-aged, out-of-shape old lady was going to tag along with Mr. Universe for an exercise demonstration. Humiliation overtook me. I was just deciding how to get out of there when Marie appeared.

She was a lovely young woman with a warm and engaging smile—truly beautiful, but not the least bit intimidating. She approached Mr. Universe and me and introduced herself. Mr. Universe was also warm and friendly. These two young people turned out to be just a few years older than my older daughter. Instead of feeling badly about that, I began to relax. They didn't act shocked that I wanted to begin to work out, and they didn't laugh at my appearance.

I began to relax as we walked upstairs to the weight room. But the next event was truly horrifying: Marie pulled out a torturous looking contraption to measure body fat!

I had not counted on this. But she assured me that it was information worth knowing and would allow her to make suggestions for productive workouts. The young man, who I'll call Tom, also seemed uncomfortable with this humiliation. He had suffered a job-related injury and was out of shape—for him. We both laughed nervously at the sight of the "fat meter," sucked in our stomachs, and let Marie do her prescribed chore.

The little pinching tool grabbed at the flabby skin on my arm, stomach, thigh, and calf. After several mathematical calculations, Marie filled out an extensive chart on each of us. Tom and I chatted as Marie figured out our body fat percentage. When she was done, she graciously and quietly told each of us how much fat we needed to lose.

The rest of the hour was spent on exercise machines. Because Tom still couldn't exercise his injured back, Marie had me try all of them. And a funny thing happened after following her instructions: I started to have fun. She didn't overtax me, and Tom was more concerned about his own rehabilitation than he was about me. I stopped thinking so much about myself and enjoyed the remaining time.

At the end of the session, Marie mentioned that she did personal training if either of us might be interested. I almost dismissed her statement, but something caused me to question her further. I had always had an image of a person who used a personal trainer as being very self-obsessed with appearance. I also thought the cost would be prohibitive.

Marie explained that the package the health club offered was a set of twelve personal training sessions that would be half the cost of taking them one at a time. The cost was $20.00 per session, with costs varying from club to club. I told her I would think about it and let her know.

I did think about it. It would be an investment in

money and time, and I couldn't change my mind. It would require a firm commitment. I thought about some things I could do without in order to justify that kind of money on personal training. Steve and I talked about it, and I prayed about it. I decided to do it.

That decision changed my failure in the exercise arena to success. I took my twelve sessions over a three-month period. Marie also worked up an exercise program for me to follow when I am traveling. I had asked her to give me something I could do in a hotel room. Marie picked out three-pound weights for me to take and had made out a chart for upper and lower body exercises.

I was away from home for six days, and I worked out with my weights every other day. I can't tell you how good I felt. I worked out in the morning before dressing for the day. It was convenient, private, and fulfilling.

Since then, I have actually gotten in the habit of working out in exercise rooms of hotels—not caring about how I look to other people. I just go and have fun. If a hotel doesn't have an exercise room, I use my weights (I'm up to five-pound weights now) in my room. Every other day for thirty minutes is all it takes.

Finding That Sense of Well-being

Not everyone can retain a personal trainer. It is costly in both time and money. But fitness is such a trend now, there are numerous at-home programs and inexpensive clubs that offer many varying ways to design a workout program that will work for you.

Weight-bearing exercises can help prevent osteoporosis and help you feel wonderful. Another kind of exercise that is beneficial is aerobic exercise to strengthen the heart. Since osteoporosis and heart disease are important concerns of menopausal women, these two kinds of exercise are wonderful additions to your health regimen.

For aerobic exercise a step aerobic program is ideal. (My husband gave me mine for Christmas.) There are several brands of equipment and the least expensive works fine. They start at about $35.00 and can be purchased in most sporting goods stores. I use two different videos that take from thirty to forty-five minutes and provide a great aerobic workout.

An ideal program is to do my step aerobics at home two to three days a week and then go to the gym for weight-bearing exercise three times a week (or use weights at home). Even if I don't get the aerobic workout in, I try to maintain the weight training three times a week.

Exercise is still very much a discipline for me, competing for my time with a myriad of other things. I still have to psych myself up to put the time in. But I *always* feel better for having done it.

That sense of well-being is not unfounded. Wulf Utian and Ruth Jacobowitz explain how exercise helps enhance mood as well as benefit the body physically:

> Exercise offers emotional benefit as well as physical energy by altering your state of mood. This alteration probably occurs because exercise activates the release of certain hormones within the brain that we call the *central endorphins* or *brain morphines*. They produce that special sense of well-being that we experience after exercise.[2]

I had started, and stopped, then started and stopped exercising more times than I can count. This time, I finally hung in with it long enough to feel results that are worth the effort.

In the past, perhaps you have decided to exercise to lose weight. This time, try thinking in terms of overall better health. Consider trying again. After you reach mid-life, you need to think of exercise as a life-long investment, not just a short-term way to shed pounds. Check ads in the newspaper for specials on membership at health clubs. Talk to women you know who exercise. Ask a friend to join you in this new endeavor and be accountable to each other. This is a way to give your body the best possible advantages as it ages.

I know. You don't want to hear another word about exercise.

Just think about it.

CHAPTER 9

....

RELAXATION BREAKS

....

*I*t is amazing to me that we as Americans can't seem to figure out how to slow down. I don't know anyone who really does a great job of living at a reasonable pace. Young, old, it doesn't matter—we are a driven people. We read books on how to relax, and we manage to alter our lifestyles for about two weeks. Most of the women interviewed in focus groups were as busy at mid-life as they were when they were thirty. They are doing different tasks, but at the same frantic pace.

But often the onset of menopause demands an adjustment. Our bodies are changing so dramatically that they can't continue to carry us speeding along in the fast lane like they used to. The time comes to intentionally take relaxation breaks.

The Warmth of the Sun

We live in Colorado, and our house sits on the crest of a hill that is seven thousand feet above sea level. Our back deck is unshaded and looks out onto the magnificent front range of the Rocky Mountains. Pikes Peak rises majestically above her court of smaller mountains to pierce the crystal blue sky in this sunny part of the country.

My idea of perfect relaxation is to sit in a lawn chair on the deck and bask in the warmth of brilliant sunshine. It is exquisitely calming to me to sit quietly and feel the sun's rays spill over my body, covering it with pleasurable penetrating heat.

I didn't use sunscreen until a few years ago, and I am afraid, to some degree, I have paid the price. My once-even tan has been replaced by sun-spotted wrinkles. So I use sunscreen now. It definitely slows the tanning process but still doesn't take away the wonderful sensation of resting in a sun-drenched world.

If you don't live in a part of the country where the sun shines a lot, don't try to re-create the same experience with a tanning booth. Besides damaging your skin it just isn't the same as being outside in God's beauty. Wait for summer days to indulge in this rejuvenating pastime.

But when summer comes, put on your sunscreen and take a sun-soaking break. It will warm your soul.

A Hot Soak in the Tub

Bubble baths do not require sunshine. They do not even have to be relegated to the evening hours of the day, although that is usually when time allows for such luxury. A shower in the morning is invigorating, but a bath at night can soothe the stress away.

If you are not so enamored of the water, consider taking a bubble bath every few weeks. Candles and classical music are wonderful additions as stress relaxers. There are countless kinds of bubbles, salts, crystals, and oils to add to bathwater, and candles come in equally numerous scents, sizes, and shapes. Some special bath promotion packages even come with floating candles to place right in the water with you. If you don't add oil to the bath water, do use body lotion after each water experience to keep your skin from looking like an alligator's.

Once in the tub, let your mind relax with your body. Think over the events of the day leisurely, or simply let your mind wander. You may find yourself praying automatically. What a peaceful time, and what soothing refreshment afterward.

The Art of Catnapping

I have a friend who used to be an accomplished catnapper. He was able to complete very long, productive days because he could nap almost anywhere.

One morning he had to take his wife to work very early. Knowing he would be tired later if he didn't nap, he grabbed a pillow from their sofa on his way out the door, and once at the office stretched out on the floor with his pillow. With the light off and the blinds drawn, he fell asleep right away. A little later his secretary came into work, right on time. Entering his office in a most businesslike fashion to turn on the light, she stumbled over his sleeping body. The dear woman thought he had had a heart attack and almost had one herself.

Sleeping in the middle of the office floor at pre-dawn hours is not recommended, but an ability to catch short naps is an asset in getting through long and stressful days.

Because menopause often drains a woman's energy, anything that can add an energy boost is helpful. Short naps—about fifteen minutes—are optimal. One friend lies down on her bed fully dressed every afternoon for just fifteen to twenty minutes. Then, she is up again and ready to go.

A key may be stretching out completely to rest. It is difficult to relax completely with the head up. Stretching the body out completely will permit total relaxation and provides a refreshing energy boost in the middle of often frantic days.

Time with a Friend

Women have been teased for years about spending hours talking on the phone. The teasing has often come from men who spend all of their days on the phone in noisy offices and can't imagine why anyone would choose to spend any additional time with the instrument.

Many women, by the time they reach the mid-life years, are working outside the home. They probably do not experience the isolation that can occur during child-rearing years, but neither are they finding meaningful interaction with others during the course of a work day.

Calling a friend does not have to take long. It can simply be a moment in the middle of the day when one woman connects with another, providing encouragement for both parties. Sometimes the unpredictability that surrounds menopause is diffused just by talking to a sympathetic listener about how you feel.

One of my dearest friends, Loretta, is a nurse. She and I talk several times a week while we are each fixing dinner. Both of our husbands arrive home late, so we take advantage of a few moments at the end of our days to touch base. Loretta is younger than I am so she is not experiencing menopause yet. But she is a sensitive listener, and her nursing background gives her insight into medical issues that I don't have.

Don't panic if your personal phone directory has no names with RN behind them. You don't need a medical professional—just a trusted friend to bring life back into perspective. Our lives are often so rushed that we can be isolated in a crowd. We may never find the close relationships our mothers enjoyed where they found them, with neighbors talking over the backyard fence while hanging laundry. A phone call can replace that loss of intimacy.

Dee, a single mother, summarized the benefits of shared time-outs. "I am so impressed by the sense that, at some level, all of us know how hard it is for women to do all they can do because of how much is demanded of them. [Friends] have been so generous of heart and spirit to help me. It raised in me a great desire to pass on some of that generosity to other women."

Feeding Our Spirits

Blank books are a popular consumer item. Any large bookstore will have a section that shelves a variety of these artistically encased blank sheets of paper designed for writing intimate thoughts. Of course, the more practical choose to use an inexpensive spiral notebook to journal. But whatever the outside cover, journals house our deepest, most precious thoughts.

A friend of mine has been journaling for over ten years and has asked me to promise that when she dies, I will retrieve her journals and dispose of them, unread. She writes her journals in the form of letters to God, and she pours her heart out openly to Him. They are for her alone, and that is the purpose of most journaling— a safe and private way to express deepest thoughts and feelings.

I don't address my journal entries to God, but I do

include prayer lists in my journal. I also jot down two categories of thoughts to help me see how God has moved me from anxiousness to peace: *On my heart* and *Peace.* I ask myself, *What am I worried about?* I write down whatever comes to mind under *On my heart.* Then I think about what feels settled and secure to me and write that down under *Peace.*

As time goes by, I can glance back at these two category entries and see how my anxious feelings have been resolved. Life doesn't always turn out the way I hoped, but I am able to see more clearly how the Lord moved through a situation and changed my anxiety into understanding, or action, or acceptance.

Chronicling the Faithfulness of God

Just a year ago a dramatic example of that process filled the pages of my journal. My son-in-law, Craig, was then a junior in college with a promising career in professional baseball well within his grasp. He was a left-handed pitcher who was being recruited by a number of professional teams. The letters and phone calls were pouring in. He and my daughter Lara were planning a December date for their wedding based on Craig being drafted by a team that June.

Then Craig started to have terrible pain in his left shoulder. He continued to play, ignoring the pain, until he could no longer deny that something was wrong. They called to tell us that he was going to the doctor. Under *On my heart* I wrote, *Worried about Craig's shoulder.*

The next day they called back with the news that the doctor, after looking at X rays, thought Craig might have a cyst or tumor. My heart sank. The word *tumor* made it to the pages of my journal. The days between

Craig having an MRI (another form of X ray) taken and the results being given were agony. In fact, during that time I couldn't even write anything under *Peace* in my journal.

Craig, gratefully, did not have a tumor. The doctor told him that what he had seen on the X ray turned out to be a bone spur, which had significantly torn up the tendons in his left arm. I was overwhelmed with thankfulness that his life was not in danger. That day, the journal entry of *Worried about Craig's shoulder* moved from *On my heart* to *Peace—Craig does not have a tumor*.

Of course, the next months were emotionally difficult for Craig and Lara as they adjusted to his baseball career being over before it began. That adjustment became a new topic in my journal where, again, I could see God moving through a difficult situation and answering prayer after prayer. Craig and Lara were married in December of 1993 and are happily pursuing careers based on Craig's interest and skill in a completely different arena than baseball.

I sometimes look back in my journal and more clearly remember the goodness of God in their lives. Those journal entries shine a light on the process from anxiousness to peace. They are a written confirmation of a passage written by Paul:

> Be anxious for nothing, but in everything by prayer and supplication, with thanksgiving, let your requests be made known to God; and the peace of God, which surpasses all understanding, will guard your hearts and minds through Christ Jesus (Phil. 4:6–7).

What we write down doesn't matter as much as the fact that we write. It is a matter of reflection. I often think I have a sense of God speaking to me or prompting me to ponder something. If I don't write it down, I may lose it. Other times, I sense insight to some matter and know that I need to sit and think through what I am sensing. Journaling helps me think things through.

Even if we only make journal entries infrequently, they can serve to unravel the tangle of changes pulsing through our lives. Write anything. It is for you and God. He can handle whatever you write. He may even use it as a way to allow you to hear Him more clearly.

Bible Reading and Prayer

As committed Christians we have all been taught to have devotions. Most of us probably read the Bible daily, and for many people prayer is like breathing. These disciplines feed our spirit. They can also provide a needed anchor in times of chaos and distressing physical symptoms. Even if they don't take the symptoms away, they can provide the stability to know that we are not alone, even in this changing time of life.

But many seasoned Christian women told others in their focus groups that their time with the Lord felt flat during menopause. They didn't leave their devotion times feeling any better than when they began them. They didn't always have the enthusiasm they used to have for Bible reading and prayer.

"My spiritual resources were powerless," Carol said. "I had always been able to draw on the Lord in times of stress, but when the emotional attacks I experienced came, it didn't work."

Other women agreed with Carol that they felt like they were groping in the dark for what previously had been readily available. These women realized that their spiritual fog was another symptom of learning to cope with both physical and physiological changes.

They understood the value of continuing in Bible reading and prayer, even if they couldn't always feel the emotions that preserved their spirits.

Meditation

While most of us are very familiar with how to read the Bible and pray, we may be novices at meditation. In fact, the very term may conjure up negative feelings. I am not suggesting meditation in any way like the New Age practice. Richard Foster, in his book *Celebration of Discipline*, explains the difference:

> All Eastern forms of meditation stress the need to be-come detached from the world. There is an emphasis upon losing personhood and individuality and merging with the Cosmic Mind. . . . Personal identity is lost in a pool of cosmic consciousness. . . . Detachment is the final goal of Eastern religion.
>
> Christian meditation goes far beyond the notion of detachment . . . we must go on to *attachment*. The de-tachment from the confusion all around us is in order to have a richer attachment to God and to other human beings.[1]

I don't practice meditation regularly or in a very structured way. I do my own thing. And my own thing is very simple. I take the phone off the hook. I sit in our sunroom at the back of the house, surrounded by win-dows and breathtaking views of the mountains. I read a short passage of Scripture, close my eyes, and wait. I sit there for a few minutes and focus on the words I've read.

Sometimes I am impressed by something very specific. One morning I was sitting with my eyes closed enjoying the warmth of the sun and thinking on the words *Christ's love*. For a few days prior to this time, I had been concerned about whether I would ever know anything about my heritage. I had only known about my adoption for about a year and had no specific information. While focusing on the words *Christ's love* I was strongly impressed with the thought that I didn't need to worry at all about finding out about my past. The Lord would reveal what He wanted me to know in due time. I could almost hear God say, "I love you and will tell you details about your past. Don't worry."

Sometimes I am not impressed with any specific thought. But there is still a sense of connection with God and a peacefulness that I seldom experience elsewhere in the hectic pace of life.

An example of a passage I like to meditate upon is Ephesians 3:14–19:

> For this reason I bow my knees to the Father of our Lord Jesus Christ, from whom the whole family in heaven and earth is named, that He would grant you, according to the riches of His glory, to be strengthened with might through His Spirit in the inner man, that Christ may dwell in your hearts through faith; that you, being rooted and grounded in love, may be able to comprehend with all the saints what is the width and length and depth and height—to know the love of Christ which passes knowledge; that you may be filled with all the fullness of God.

When I sit in my sunroom, with the majesty of the Rocky Mountains before me, and think quietly on this passage, I am overwhelmed. I am struck with how incomprehensible is the love of God. I leave from moments like those with a reassurance that I really am loved far more than I can imagine. It is renewing.

Another Scripture passage that equally provides many days of meditation suggestions is Philippians 4:8:

> Finally, brethren, whatever things are true, whatever things are noble, whatever things are just, whatever things are pure, whatever things are lovely, whatever things are of good report, if there is any virtue and if there is anything praiseworthy—meditate on these things.

Dream Again

"What are your dreams?" I asked one focus group.

"Things don't thrill me like they used to," Nancy replied. She once had had dreams that excited her, but she hadn't thought about them for years.

Penny expressed similar feelings. "I don't have a big desire to do too much. I feel kind of lazy."

We talked about how it is so hard to figure out "what I want to be when I grow up." When we were young we could dream more enthusiastically because we still had lots of time to accomplish our dreams. For some of us, our dreams were focused on raising our children with little attention to what we might dare attempt after they were grown.

I have always loved the verse, "Therefore we also, since we are surrounded by so great a cloud of witnesses, let us lay aside every weight, and the sin which so easily ensnares us, and let us run with endurance the race that is set before us" (Heb. 12:1).

But when my younger daughter left home, I found I had no finish line in view for the race I was to run. I couldn't decide what God wanted me to do or what

I thought I could do. I still have moments when the ribbon across the finish line is blurred. Discouragement comes when I feel too old to pursue dreams.

It's Not Too Late

I remember being in a seminar where Florence Littauer was the keynote speaker. She gave a talk based on her book *Silver Boxes: The Gift of Encouragement*. It is a wonderful story about her father who didn't accomplish some of his dreams because of a lack of encouragement. But he gave the gift of encouragement to Florence. In another one of her books, *Dare to Dream*, she says,

> I try to give each one hope by saying, "It's never too late to dare to dream. I didn't write my first book until I was almost fifty. Get moving!" I'm convinced from the overwhelming response I've received from *Silver Boxes* that almost everyone has a latent desire within them that has not been fulfilled.[2]

I have always been a big dreamer. But I must agree with some of the women in the focus groups. It is harder to be excited about new endeavors in the midst of mid-life circumstances and difficult symptoms of menopause.

I have spent many hours in bed before drifting off to sleep thinking about the future and the pursuit of meaningful dreams. One thought that comes back to me over and over again is that when I feel good physically, I feel enthusiastic about running a new race. But when I feel bad physically, I don't feel like doing anything. I am convinced that once the physical symptoms of menopause are over, there is a renewed vision for life.

For those of us in the middle of the process, we need to hang on during the tough part.

That is one reason why I find that taking a few quiet minutes to think about the future is comforting—and even exciting. I allow my mind to wonder:

If I could do anything at all and be sure of success, what would I do?

The answer that most often comes to my mind is that I would love to write and speak with such power that teeming masses would read or hear my words and their lives would be changed. They would be sincerely encouraged about themselves and their lives, and they would be enticed to long for an intimate relationship with Jesus. In my dreams, my books sell millions and I speak to stadium-filled audiences.

Reality hasn't caught up with my dreams yet, but I am drawn on by the image of a future in which I continue to run the race set before me.

What is your dream?

Something Bubbling

When I found my primary role in life changing from parent to parent-of-adult-children, I suffered a sense of loss and confusion. But I also felt a bubbling excitement pushing its way up into my consciousness. In the middle of all the frustrations and choices of mid-life, there was an exuberant, inner urging to reach back and play with some long-ago forsaken treasures.

For me, this play results in pockets of time where I enjoy life for the sheer joy of it. I sit and play the piano, even though I really can't play. I fiddle with the familiar pieces I know and don't worry about perfecting them for anyone else to hear. I ride up into the mountains and eat lunch at a quaint Swiss restaurant and remember wonderful trips to other countries. I go to a local coffeehouse where a lot of college students hang out and pretend I'm in a Paris café. And I am planning to ice skate again. I loved to skate growing up and dreamed of being an Olympic competitor. I haven't skated in over eight years, and now I just want to put my old skates on to see how they feel. I feel no pressure to be a champion, only a desire to enjoy the sound of the blade on the ice and remember many happy times.

Julia Cameron, in her book *The Artist's Way* talks about this reviving of our creative energies:

> We begin to excavate our buried dreams. This is a tricky process. Some of our dreams are very volatile, and the mere act of brushing them off sends an enormous surge of energy bolting through our denial system. Such grief! Such loss! Such pain! . . . We mourn the self we abandoned.[3]

But what joy to dabble in pursuits that delight our souls. I know several women who have begun to do just that. One has begun to paint again after over twenty years. She paints for her own enjoyment and pleasure. Another has started a class in a foreign language. Others write poetry, pick up a discarded musical instrument and play again, read extensively on a topic of interest just for the fun of it, or embark on a host of other adventures.

The Presence of God

None of these pursuits are antithetical to the pursuit of God. Of course, any of them could be misused and turned into a barrier to seeking God. But I have found that I often see God more clearly when I allow myself this kind of free-spirited play, for my spiritual insight is sharpened.

When I ride up to the mountains, I see God's benediction all around me. Gliding across the floor of an ice rink transports me to a place of physical freedom where the hindrances to movement fall off and I soar. In those moments, my soul soars too.

So often, in seeking God, we limit our search to the known and routine. We segregate our spiritual lives into the times we are reading the Bible, praying, or attending church. There is great spiritual reality in enjoying life in ways that express ourselves as God has made us. We don't abandon the known and routine.

We become more balanced. Most of us are pretty tightly wound and fearful of being too frivolous. The second half of life can become so much more joyful if we launch out a little. We don't move away from God in that launching out. He comes with us and gives us the incredible riches of His grace to enjoy His world and our existence in it.

....

CHAPTER 10

I DON'T WANT TO TALK TO MEN ABOUT MENOPAUSE

....

I didn't want to interview any men for this book.

"Are you kidding?" I responded when my male publisher said he wanted a section on what men think about menopause.

"I already know what men think," I protested.

Men think menopausal women are powder kegs about to explode at the least jostle. Men make jokes about women aging and being hysterical and looking awful and forgetting their own names and sweating buckets and talking in rambling sentences. . . .

My mind flashed back to an encounter I had had with a male friend. I was sitting on the floor of a local Christian bookstore, looking through the women's section to see what was already published on menopause, when I heard a familiar voice say, "Lois, is that you?"

I looked up to see Tony, the husband of a woman I know.

"Hi, Tony!"

"What are you up to?" he asked. "You look pretty intent."

"Oh," I said as I got up from my studious position. "I'm doing a book and checking out what's already been written on the subject."

"What's the book about?" he asked.

"Well," I replied, lowering my voice so no one else could hear, "it's about women and mid-life." I couldn't bring myself to utter the word *menopause*.

I couldn't believe it. He blushed. He shuffled, he looked down, and finally he said, "Lois, if you write a book on *that*, you'll end up going around the country *talking* about it."

Tony changed the subject and we stayed on safe topics until it seemed natural for him to leave. As soon as he was out of sight, I turned and hurried out of the store.

I felt ashamed. Ashamed! Why did I feel like I had done something shameful? His response seemed to verify what I thought I knew about how men think about menopause—it's too embarrassing to even talk about.

Webster defines *shame* as "a painful feeling of having lost the respect of others because of the improper behavior, incompetence, of oneself or another." I think women feel like their behavior during menopause causes men to lose respect for them. They believe they are seen as frantic females who cannot control themselves.

I argued with my publisher that all women, not just me, knew what men thought. He persisted. Steve agreed with him. They outnumbered me.

Men, I thought sullenly. *What do they know about how women feel about this touchy subject? Why would women want to read about the jokes the men are telling?*

What Husbands Say

I thought about getting together a focus group in the same way I had interviewed women, but I was nervous about calling these men and explaining the concept of a group of men getting together to talk about menopause.

So I called one of the more sensitive men that I know. He is a counselor and natural encourager. He and his wife are in their late forties, so I thought he would have the contacts with men in the right age group. Paul was wonderful. He agreed to get about ten guys together at his house for an evening group that I would facilitate. The only requirement for these men was that their wives had started to have some of the symptoms of menopause.

The day of the group meeting arrived, and I almost called it off. I felt really vulnerable at the thought of me and all these men talking about the "M" word. The wives had decided to gather at another house while I interviewed their husbands. When I arrived at Paul's, I was grateful that his wife and a few of the other wives were still there. But as they left, I felt more strongly than ever that I should be going with them instead of staying with the men.

Despite my apprehension, the evening was great. The men were kind, comfortable, and eager to help. I began by asking them how they felt about what their wives were going through.

Mike

Mike, who was the oldest, began with an admission that he had not been very sensitive when his wife had gone through menopause.

"I was a fifties kind of guy in a nineties setting," he

said. "I remember not being very aware of what was going on."

Mike's wife is past menopause now, so his presence at the meeting was an encouragement to the other men. The rest of them expressed knowing very little, or thinking very little, about menopause before their wives had started to display early symptoms.

Ted

Ted, whose wife has very few symptoms, said that he was apprehensive about his wife entering menopause because of what he had heard years ago in college. He had a professor who told his classes that his wife went through the change and divorced him. Ted admitted that he had no other information on menopause.

Scott

Scott said that he really had no idea what to expect either as his wife began to have some symptoms. The only thing he has noticed so far is that his wife was nervous about her loss of memory.

"I told her," Scott said, "I must have been going through menopause for the last ten years—my memory is gone.

"I want to be supportive, but I really don't know what to say. I want to be an authority, but I am not."

Dwayne

Dwayne sat listening to the other men talk with pensive interest. He told the group that he and his wife are on the front part of being there with a capital "T." *There* describes mid-life with all of its changes—retirement, new job, kids leaving, physical changes for him and his wife.

"I don't feel very attached to her problem," Dwayne said, referring to his wife's decisions on how to handle menopausal symptoms, "which is strange for me. I am more intrigued and fascinated with what is happening to my eternally youthful wife and the impact that is going to have at a time of transition in my own life."

Dwayne went on to tell how he has learned to recognize when his wife wants to be left alone. He knows that she means nothing against him, but he feels she wants to handle her feelings in her own way.

Several men agreed with Dwayne that they feel like spectators. They watch and care, but don't know what to do. Menopause is perceived as a women's issue, so they tend to let their wives figure out what to do about how they feel.

Matt

Matt had been divorced before his current marriage and feels he learned a lot the first time around. His first wife, though not at the age of menopause, had emotional mood swings. When she did, Matt would detach because he felt hurt and beat up. Now, in his current marriage, he feels he better understands the role emotions play in menopause. He and his wife have been able to connect emotionally. He attributes that connection to his experience in his first marriage, his increased knowledge as a result of becoming a counselor, and his wife's ability to handle difficulties well.

Paul

"I think there is a correlation between menopause for women and hair loss for men," Paul said as he ran his hand over his smooth, shiny head. A few other comments about waistline bulges confirmed that these men were beginning to experience their own mid-life symptoms.

Paul continued, "I think we don't talk about menopause because it has to do with sex. There is a taboo in talking about it."

Paul is also a counselor and talks to a lot of women who are suffering from menopausal symptoms. He said he tries to be supportive of them and encourages them to speak up. He thinks the public needs to be educated so that women with symptoms will get them checked out.

New Ideas and New Experiences

Surprisingly, the men in this focus group were as comfortable and supportive as the women had been. Their comments reflected how the topic had opened up some new thoughts for them:

Dwayne: "My attitudes are that it is her [my wife] going through this passage and I view me as stationary. And yet, when I look at it realistically I realize I am *there*. There is a solemnity in me. Proof to me that we are in another season of life. This is serious stuff."

Matt: "I think it has to do with nurturing. When our wives are ill, we need to be nurturing, and these are not natural things for us. God has really been putting us [husbands] through some maturing and growing so we can be there for them at this stage of life."

Scott: "It is a real learning process for women. Emotions are high, but it is because of going through menopause, retirement, empty nest. There is a lot going on. Women try to compare with other women."

Paul: "The problem is when we make comparisons, it is a criticism. Part of my anger is that when we go through stages we don't deal very well with losses.

When society values youth and values women for beauty and childbearing, I think women need support. I bought a plaque when we moved here, *Come grow old with me, the best is yet to be*. It really should be that way—trying to be sensitive about losses."

Paul's comments about beauty and comparison led to a discussion about the pressure put on women to remain physically attractive. One of the men said that he and his wife enjoy wonderful, intimate times and that she is still very sexually attractive to him. But she worries about having put on a few pounds and not looking like a model.

They agreed that the loss of physical beauty is difficult and that they want to be affirming and encouraging to their wives. They admitted that seeing their wives deal with physical changes caused them to think more about their own aging process.

"I can't run as far or as fast as I used to. My hair is thinning. My waist is thicker," Paul said as the others nodded their heads in agreement.

"I can't read a thing without my glasses," someone else said.

"I am winded much quicker than I used to be," Matt added.

Someone finally ventured a question about sex after menopause. "What will happen down the road sexually to my wife? Will we end up in separate bedrooms? Some of you are *there*. What's it like?"

"If people are loving and communicating," Paul answered, "things are fine."

Someone else chimed in that you might not continue to have sex as frequently, which caused Mike (the menopause veteran in the group) to grin broadly. Then the rest of the group started to grin, as if to say it had been some years since most of them had been as sexually active as in their youth. No one else said anything more, but they seemed content to trust that their wives would not be moving out of their bedrooms.

Dwayne summarized the sentiment in the room by the end of the evening. "I wish we had had this conversation five years ago. I have learned more from my peers than I could have imagined. I would not talk like this on the golf course or anywhere. Has anyone ever heard a man mention that his wife is going through menopause? Never. Men don't talk about it and it is so helpful. What I have concluded is that I shouldn't be so passive as I am now and pay more attention to what my wife is going through. I'm going to encourage discussion and share myself more."

As I folded up my laptop to head for home, someone eagerly asked, "What do they say about us? What do they want us to do?"

And that is the subject of the next chapter.

CHAPTER 11

....

WHAT WIVES WISH THEIR HUSBANDS KNEW

....

*M*en want to fix everything," one woman told her group. "I just want him to hold me and tell me he still loves me."

Her sentiments ring true for many women. There is no easy fix. What women want is to know that their husbands will stay connected to them, or begin connecting with them, and ride through this stage of life together.

"Don't give a lot of advice," another woman responded when asked about what she tells her husband she needs. "I want to be able to say how I feel without feeling like I have to take his advice."

This woman may sound ungrateful, but she is only frustrated. It is difficult for men to accept that there is nothing they can do to make menopausal symptoms go away. But wives do think there is a lot that husbands can do to be supportive.

Understand that emotional symptoms are (usually) caused by physiological changes, not by husbands.

One woman said, "My husband never knows exactly what he'll find when he gets home from work. Some

131

days I am my normal self, which is pretty calm. Other days, I am off the wall. I am agitated and tearful. He comes in and I just light right into him. I don't mean to take my frustration out on him, but I do."

Other women talked about how they want their husbands to understand that they are not the cause of emotional outbursts. But they may be the recipients of this symptom. It does seem to be asking a lot to expect men to bear the brunt of fluctuating emotions without taking it personally. But if husbands take emotional mood swings at face value, they may be hurt in ways their wives never intended.

Steve and I have talked about how to get through the times I feel like an emotional basket case. He tries not to be detached but to verbalize that he is sorry I feel badly and is there for me. I try to remember that this feeling is not caused by him, and it will pass. He doesn't pressure me to change, and most importantly, I allow myself some time alone to regain my composure.

Of course, couples can have interpersonal problems that cause emotional distress completely unrelated to menopause. There may be stress over adjusting to issues such as children leaving home, caring for elderly parents, finances, and retirement. These issues need to be addressed with reference to whatever is the root cause of the problem—communication, self-worth, and more.

Don't make fun of menopausal women.

Women don't want to be the object of jokes. A sense of humor is fine, but jokes or remarks about being old or menopausal don't build relationships. It is especially painful if jokes or hurtful comments are made in front of other people. Most couples are able to laugh together privately about some of the strange behaviors women demonstrate, but only after the symptoms causing the behavior have passed. Steve and I often joke about my forgetfulness, but privately and not at the moment I am frantically looking for a vanished item.

Validate that symptoms are real.

In the same way that women don't want to be the objects of jokes, they do want their feelings validated. They don't want to be dismissed as hysterical or suffering from some imaginary dysfunction. They don't want to be told that their symptoms are cases of mind over matter—change your mind and the matter will change.

Men can help communicate a validation of feelings by being willing to read a book or an article that explains menopause. They don't need to be experts, but showing interest is very encouraging.

Support new interests.

Many women are venturing out into new territory during the mid-life years. They may be going back to work for the first time in years, going back to school, or picking up an old interest with new enthusiasm. It is wonderful to be asked about any new area with sincere interest. These conversations are not unlike the dinner conversations where men talk about their time at work. Women are encouraged when their husband remembers and is willing to spend time talking about her interests.

Some men may need to adjust their own schedules to accommodate their wife's schedules. Maybe dinner will be a pizza from the local take-out instead of a home cooked meal because a wife takes a class two days a week that doesn't end until six o'clock.

Remain faithful.

There are all too many stories of men who leave their wives during mid-life crises. This term is often used to explain why men become involved with younger women.

An article in *Woman's Day* quoted a rise in percentage of divorces after the age of fifty-five due, in part, to this very reason:

> They enter their golden years and their husband walks out the door, often for a younger woman. That's what's happening to an increasing number of women in their fifties and sixties these days. While divorce among younger people seems to be leveling off, there's a worrisome rise in marriage breakups among the over-fifty-five crowd—up 22 percent in the last decade and expected to climb.[1]

These women must grapple with their own feelings of low self-esteem and inadequacy. Most women I interviewed privately said that they didn't know of their husband's feelings which led to the affairs until it was too late. The husband had met whatever needs they had superficially in relationships with other women.

Mid-life can be a rough time for both men and women, but a solid commitment to weather the storms together will help solve problems. Unfaithfulness by either men or women will only create many more painful problems.

Ask questions, really listen, and respond.

Women want their husbands to talk to them. They want their husbands to risk asking them how they feel. Husbands might encounter differing responses to that question—emotional reactions, withdrawals, confusion, appreciative answers—but, whatever the response, most women appreciate interest in how they feel.

"My problem," Marie said, "is that my husband will ask me how I feel, then he won't really listen to what I say. He asks me as he is walking into the other room, or glancing at the paper, or shuffling through the mail. So I answer and that is the end of the conversation. His question was not sincere."

The helpful sequence goes like this: Ask, listen, respond. For those husbands who say they don't know how to respond, it's okay to say, "I don't know what to say, but I want to try to understand."

Women want to know they are cared for and cared about. They want to know that their husbands think about them. And for women, that means verbal interaction.

The Challenging Mix of Dating and Menopause

Thus far the focus of this discussion has been on men and women who are still married to each other. But many women find themselves single—or single again—and "available" during the menopause years.

I know from personal experience that dating as an adult can be the pits. Add the onset of menopause and it can be a calamity. Imagine being with a man you find attractive and suddenly you're sweating into your shrimp cocktail. Or his asking you what happened at work that day, and you can't remember. Of course, there's always the threat of the appearance of a thirty-year-old female knockout to push you over the edge and into an anxiety attack.

And heaven forbid if you have an unexplained mood swing in the middle of a first date. You may have sealed your fate with that man forever. If husbands have tough times understanding wives they have lived with for decades, imagine the inability of the dating males to be charming in the face of menopause.

"My last date was a real nightmare," Rhonda proclaimed. "There was no seat on the passenger side of his car, and I had to move fishing poles to get in the back seat."

Rhonda, full of humor and drama, painted a picture of an evening spent listening to her date complaining about the cost of every item on the menu of the restaurant he had selected. When he wasn't complaining, he was talking about himself. Then when he dropped her off at her house he began to talk about wanting to get married and have children.

Rhonda is in her late forties and has had a hysterectomy.

"It was the first time I mourned the loss of my parts," she said to an already smiling group of women. With her reference to "parts," we all broke into roars of laughter, including Rhonda.

Her disappointing date was worsened by the reality that she wasn't young enough to provide what many men want. This particular man would, undoubtedly, not have been a marriage candidate for Rhonda even if she had been much younger. But his desire for children isn't all that uncommon.

Many single women are able to listen to dating war stories like Rhonda's and laugh because they are past the game-playing stage. Most of them accept themselves and are not interested in trying to become what a man wants. They are themselves and, if they meet men who appreciate them for who they are, great. If not, they are not willing to try to be someone else's fantasy.

Single middle-aged men are in a tough spot, too. They have their own pains and issues of mid-life to handle in addition to deciding how to relate to women. Successful dating relationships in the mid-life years seem to depend on the maturity of the people involved. Mature men and women can enjoy meaningful relationships if they are able to be themselves and accept others as they are also.

Feelings of Threatened Sexuality

Women who are grappling with signs of physical aging often feel like their very sexuality is threatened. They think they are not viewed as *sexy*, but often they don't even feel sexual anymore. Our culture tangles sexuality—the comprehensive quality of femininity or masculinity—with sexiness—the erotic quality of arousing sexual desire. It is important to see the distinction.

God created Eve female and she remained female all of her life. She didn't reach mid-life and suddenly turn into a neuter life form. We who are born female remain female until we die. Our sexuality continues to be expressed throughout our lives. Certainly the end of childbearing years marks a change in one expression of our sexuality. But this does not change us into nonsexual beings.

The characteristics of mid-life sexuality that Christian women in the focus groups expressed included contentment, acceptance, graciousness, kindness—those qualities that reflect a woman who understands, in some small way, what it means to be in the presence of her Creator and knows that He sees her as completely feminine, no matter what her age.

What we lose as we age is not our sexuality; it is only the physical body of youth. What the world calls *sexy* does fade away. Who we are as sexual beings remains with us all the days of our lives.

Thinking About Sexuality

One woman in the focus groups said, "I've heard that there are three stages of life: youth, mid-life, and, 'My, you're looking well.'"

We all laughed at her sarcastic reference to "looking well," and then we remembered the days when the word *well* would have meant "pretty," "beautiful," or even "fantastic." Most of us in the group had felt the sting of fading from the ranks of the physically praised and moving to the sidelines of the cosmetically concealed. The telltale compliment that marks the move from physically attractive to showing one's age is, *You are looking great, for a woman your age.*

Living in a society that so worships physical, sexual perfection, it is difficult to change our thinking from placing great value on physical appeal to placing that value on inner beauty. Things are a little better than they were a decade ago: Women are valued for more than winning beauty contests; some are moving into high-ranking professional positions as a result of qualifications, not looks; and they are more frequently written about in magazines and newspapers for their accomplishments. But the touting of the youthful and well-built female, with big breasts, small waist, shapely hips, long legs, wrinkle-free skin, silky hair, and fat-free body, is alive.

That ideal places incredible pressure on girls and young women, but it completely slips from the realm of possibility for women moving into their forties and fifties.

The women I interviewed were at different stages in

the process of accepting physical aging and retaining healthy feelings about their sexuality. The very first group I talked with surprised me with their responses. I asked a question about the cosmetic industry targeting mid-life women with anti-aging products.

"We're too smart to fall for that kind of advertising," one woman replied.

The others agreed that they had long ago given up running after the elusive myth of the physically perfect woman. These women were enjoying a self-acceptance that proved not to be shared by many other women interviewed.

"It is just so hard to catch my reflection in a mirror and see that I am not as young as I feel I am," said Terry, an attractive woman in her late forties. "I used to get a lot of compliments on how good I looked. That doesn't happen so often anymore."

The realities of mid-life and aging—weight gain, wrinkles, sagging bodies, gray hair—may cause us to feel badly about ourselves. So how can we change our thinking about our sexuality?

We accept that we are not sexy young things. But sexuality is not about attracting men with physical beauty. It is about accepting who we are and how we look. And as we go through mid-life, our sexuality is enhanced, for we become more comfortable with ourselves in light of the physical changes in our bodies.

I really think that I am a softer person than I was a few years ago: I don't react to situations with sarcasm; I accept differing opinions more graciously. I also know that I look older; my face has more wrinkles; my waist is a little thicker. But I believe that my sexuality is more readily perceived in my softer personality than it used to be in my younger look.

Thinking about our sexuality means letting go of old images of the sexy female. It means appreciating the qualities of mature beauty that allow for a few wrinkles to surround a smile or gray hair to highlight a kind face. It also means giving men more credit than we sometimes do. Many godly men do appreciate women as they get older and respect their sexuality in godly ways. And that contributes to a woman's feeling cherished, appreciated, and worthwhile long after she's lost the world's outer trappings of beauty.

CHAPTER 12

....

LOOKING FOR
RELIEF AND POWER

....

*B*efore I talk about the spiritual aspects of mid-life, let me look back on my own spiritual foundation.

I was first introduced to Jesus at a Bible camp when I was thirteen. Sitting around the campfire on a chilly Tuesday night in August somewhere in eastern Pennsylvania, I heard that it was possible to have a relationship with God by inviting His Son into my life as my own personal Savior. The minister leading the evening service talked about forgiveness and reconciliation with God. I understood that Jesus loved me so much that He had taken the payment for my transgressions against God onto Himself. I was forgiven and completely accepted by God because of Jesus. It was the most touching message I had ever heard, and I prayed to invite this beautiful Jesus into my heart.

He came. I felt His presence that night and I have ever since. I spent many years hearing little more than the salvation invitation I had heard that night at camp. My parents were not Christians then and the church I attended didn't preach the gospel. But I never felt alone again. I felt that Jesus was with me and understood my every longing.

By my mid-twenties, I had married and become actively involved in a spiritually vibrant evangelical church. Our family grew in our knowledge of what it meant to have an authentic relationship with Christ. That faith was dramatically tested in December of 1979 when my first husband, Jack, and three other people were killed in a hot-air balloon accident. Lisa and Lara, my daughters, and I witnessed the accident along with the wife and fiancée of the two men killed with him, Rick Rhine and Glen Berg.

The shock of seeing these men die was tempered by the overwhelming reality of eternal life. God's grace that day, and in all the years since, was poured out on us and saturated us with the sweet assurance of our loved ones being in heaven. All three men had accepted Christ as Savior. Eternal life in heaven is their inheritance.

Mid-life: A Time of Spiritual Reflection

In the years since that fateful day, I have continued to experience life lived in relationship with God through faith in His Son and trust in His Holy Spirit.

But when those first early symptoms of menopause hit, something new happened. The emotional ups and downs were different from the emotional responses I had experienced in the past. I began to feel disconnected from everything that had once been familiar. My children were grown and gone. I had remarried, and my marriage was new and unfamiliar. My body was not responding as it always had. I was overwhelmed with a sense of fragmentation.

I never stopped praying or relating to God. I knew He was still active in my life. I just *felt* so strange—so distant from everyone. During that time I allowed myself to become much more open with the Lord than I ever had in the past. I expressed my frustration to Him about how I felt and asked Him questions about things I had taken for granted. I wondered about the church and its role in society. I questioned if my own heart was right toward all of God's people, including the poor and disenfranchised. Was I too comfortable in my neat little Christian circle of friends? How should I spend my time, now that my priorities had shifted from being a full-time parent?

These may seem like aimless ramblings of one hysterical woman, but many of the women interviewed in the focus groups expressed similar feelings. They were relieved to hear that other Christian women had had the same thoughts.

Menopause rocks the boat. It stirs up the emotions and results in much soul-searching. The result for me—and for many other women—has been a deeper, much more personal faith. God seems bigger. He is not only defined by doctrine and theology. He is defined by person-to-person encounters in the quiet of questioning hearts. The questions are about living lives of significance. What is truly important? What does God want us to do differently? How can we better love Him? It is a freeing time to look again at what we believe and reevaluate how to reflect the reality of Christ in our lives in unique and personal ways.

Women Seeking Spiritual Answers

Christian women are not unique in their mid-life spiritual thoughts. Many secular books and articles attest to the fact that menopause involves a spiritual dimension. These writings seek to apply spiritual remedies to relieve symptoms, inspire meaning in life, and accept death.

Over twenty million women in the U.S. alone will enter menopause in the next decade. They are beginning to read about their distressing symptoms, seek options for treatment, and look into the experiences of other women during this life-changing passage. Spirituality is a topic of great interest to many of these women. Even those who have been very pragmatic are faced with emerging thoughts of the deeper meaning of life and the prospect of death. These women are raising questions and seeking answers on a subject that they can no longer deny with cavalier existentialism.

Barbara Ehrenreich, in her article "Coming of Age," explores what feminist writers are saying about aging women and thoughts of death.

> This is not a phase that ends in marriage or a Nobel prize or promotion to branch manager (though all those things could well happen at any point). This is a phase that ends in death. Like it or not, the great spiritual task of the later years is not to be busier, prettier, or more productive than anyone else, but to be prepared for the fact of death. And this is one task, the philosophers agree, that cannot be accomplished in a condition of terminal busy-ness. . . .
>
> The fact is that we will be dead when we die—and nothing in our individualistic, competitive souls prepares us to think not just of "death," in the sense of a deadline, but of actually being dead: as in *no more me*.[1]

Popular secular books are attempting to satisfy women's mid-life quest for meaning with a mixture of medical data, nonmedical methods of treatment, and spiritual panaceas. Those spiritual prescriptions include answers to questions about meaning and power in life and acceptance of death. But are they trustworthy?

Take a look at what many women are reading as they pursue spiritual questions.

Alternative Spiritual Remedies

Gayle Sand wrote a particularly funny book about menopause entitled *Is It Hot in Here or Is It Me?* Sand has been a columnist, restaurant critic, and editor-at-large for a Florida newspaper. Her book chronicles her search for relief from ravaging hot flashes. Sand, determined not to use HRT, turned to the New Age marketplace to find a cure. Her escapades took her from acupuncture to a drink from the famed Fountain of Youth in Florida. Some of the other approaches she tried had distinctly spiritual components. One example was a visit to a spiritual healer:

> My hairdresser, Sylvie, a very spiritual vegetarian, suggested that I visit Hilda, a spiritual healer. According to Sylvie, Hilda is the real thing: "She was struck by lightning when she was three, was meditating at four, and was healing pets at five. Then they wrote her up in the *National Enquirer.*" The *Enquirer* is not exactly *The New England Journal of Medicine* but I was still impressed. I think you should get a second opinion, even with faith healers, so I asked around. I spoke to several of the healer's satisfied healees and they all said the same thing: "Let Hilda lay hands on your menopause."[2]

Hilda didn't heal Sand. None of her New Age attempts helped. She ended up taking hormones after all.

Sand presents her spiritual adventures with humor, but admitted she had been willing to try anything to find relief from her debilitating hot flashes. Had any of the New Age remedies provided the relief she sought, she probably would have practiced them willingly.

Gail Sheehy writes about spirituality in mid-life in a more serious tone. Her book, *Silent Passage*, includes a chapter entitled "Wisewoman Power" that explains her spiritual views.

> Wisdom, or the collective practical knowledge of the culture that is more simply termed common sense, has continued up through history to be associated with older women. Even in premodern times, when Christianity rejected females as deities or primary healers, great public women did emerge and exert their influence through the religious system. Some became prized as advisers to emperors and popes, turned to for their healing powers, venerated as holy—and it turns out that they were usually near fifty when they took on this aura of wisewoman.[3]

How to Respond

We have a choice in how to respond to the teaching in these, and other, popular books on menopause. We can judge and condemn women who delve into books offering non-Christian spirituality, or we can engage with them so that we have an opportunity to understand these women and impact their thinking.

We can go through this time of life focused on ourselves (admittedly, that is often all we can handle). Or we can look around us and see millions of other women in the same boat in need of true answers.

Menopausal symptoms can last for up to ten years. Most of us don't experience a nonstop need to focus on ourselves during all those years. In those moments or months of calm, we can venture out into the lives of other women and seize the opportunity for impact. If we have no idea what women outside the Christian community are reading and thinking, it is unlikely we will generate much curiosity about how a relationship with Jesus Christ changes lives and overcomes death.

As Christians, we are not to dabble in spurious, spiritual teachings of the world. I am not suggesting that we become experts on the New Age and metaphysical doctrines suggested in so many of the secular books on the market today. But maybe we need to have a better understanding of what's out there. I do think we need to be aware of the tremendous interest in spirituality and seek to present the message of the Gospels.

In reading these books I have been continually struck by a desire for spiritual truth. Even the most ardent feminists are opening the door for discussions about faith. Germaine Greer wrote a stinging book, *The Change*, which lashes out at the medical community and rallies her readers with a clarion call to denounce sexual stereotypes and grasp the power menopause produces. Near the end of this book, she actually acknowledges the potential place of traditional religion in the life of menopausal women:

> Religion is one of the easiest ways that the aging woman can unlock the door to her interior self. If she has been an unreflective Christian or Hindu or Muslim or Jew or Buddhist she may find it easier to find her interior life by entering more deeply into the implications of her religion. Examples of the piety of older women are to be seen on all sides; what is not so easy to discern is the joy that entering into the intellectual edifices of the great religions can give to those who have faith.[4]

Greer's view, like that of many secular women, is that Christianity produces little joy. Since religion holds little appeal to the unchurched, many of these women choose spiritual paths that lead them away from God and into themselves. How sad.

We, as Christian women, have much to offer women who acknowledge their spiritual thirst. We are unlikely to impact the writers of these books or leaders in non-traditional spiritual movements. But we come into daily contact with women who are buying these books.

Instead of simply dismissing these books as evil, we need to be asking ourselves, *What is the appeal of this kind of teaching? How can we have a greater influence on women buying into these methods?*

We don't have to compromise any of our own beliefs to ask these questions. We are not looking at what the secular market is saying in order to accept its doctrines ourselves.

If we find ourselves intrigued with teaching that we are tempted to embrace ourselves, we can test the spirit of the teaching. Scripture tells us the measure of the true Spirit of God:

> Beloved, do not believe every spirit, but test the spirits, whether they are of God; because many false prophets have gone out into the world. By this you know the Spirit of God: Every spirit that confesses that Jesus Christ has come in the flesh is of God, and every spirit that does not confess that Jesus Christ has come in the flesh is not of God. And this is the spirit of the Antichrist, which you have heard was coming, and is now already in the world. You are of God, little children, and have overcome them, because He who is in you is greater than he who is in the world. They are of the world. Therefore they speak as of the world, and the world hears them. We are of God. He who knows God hears us; he who is not of God does not hear us. By this

we know the spirit of truth and the spirit of error
(1 John 4:1–6).

If we remain in communion with God and His people, we will recognize error. If we are drawn to false-
hood, we need to disengage. Some women involved in
non-Christian spiritual pursuits may be trying to bring
us into their way of thinking. We have power to engage
with them for the sake of the gospel, but if we feel weak
and vulnerable, we can pull back.

When our spiritual resources are replenished, we can
lovingly move back out into dialogue with nonbelievers
and seek opportunities to impact them toward interest
in knowing Christ. While we may not have a spiritual
commonality and a common hunger for God, we have a
gender commonality. Menopause is no respecter of per-
sons. It happens to every single woman who lives long
enough. If it is a time of spiritual questioning, as it certainly seems to be, then it provides a great opportunity
for us to reflect our relationship with Christ to those
women who do not know Him.

Looking for Relief

For women experiencing distressing symptoms during menopause, first and foremost they want relief. The
Christian may look to God for immediate, physical answers. In the safety of focus groups, these women were
very honest as to what happened next.

Many of them admitted that in the early stages of
menopause they felt that their faith in Christ would get
them through any discomfort without medical intervention. Some of them felt guilty when that was not the
case.

One frustrated woman who has emotional ups and

downs said, "I should be able to overcome this. What is wrong with me? I find myself unhappy and living with uncertainty. I go to the Lord and teach Bible studies and listen to tapes, but sometimes I feel bad anyway. I get these waves of anxiety. I can be perfectly fine and a wave of fear comes."

Another woman gave an impassioned account of how she had gone from doctor to doctor to find relief for emotional stress. She had suffered from it all her life, but it worsened during menopause. None of the doctors took her seriously. Some of her Christian friends insisted she just needed to pray more and stop looking for medical help.

She ignored her friends' admonitions and finally saw a psychiatrist who diagnosed clinical depression. Her family had a history of depression and suicide. The doctor put her on antidepressant medication which she still takes. She is a committed Christian who understands that her body needs medical help in order for her to function well. She has stopped feeling guilty that her faith alone couldn't make her feel better.

While there are certainly accounts of miraculous healings, many Christians appropriately make use of medical assistance to cope with varying forms of illness. Contrary to the idea that using medicine is a cop-out, one group concluded that God gave doctors certain gifts to use in healing. One of the writers of Scripture, Luke, was a physician. They saw no contradiction of Scripture in using medical means of improving life.

Other women found great relief in their relationship with the Lord. Their experience was just the opposite of the women who didn't find relief in spiritual pursuits.

"God's Word is life and health to my flesh," Amy said.

"It [menopause] has brought me closer to the Lord. Other things that help me cope are Christian music, reading the Bible, praying, and fellowship. These things I really depend on."

As Amy talked on, she explained that the relief was not physical, but spiritual—an inner sense of well-being despite what she was feeling. She still has hot flashes and emotional distress.

"It [peace with God] coexists with the fragmentation."

Some other women felt that their spirituality was the only thing that helped them cope with menopause. When they felt overwhelmed with emotions they would go off alone and pray. They would spend quiet time with the Lord and regain composure and experience relief. Whether they felt better or not, most of the Christian women in the focus groups agreed that the spiritual comfort was crucial when dealing with the changing circumstances of mid-life.

The storms of mid-life come and go, but the peace that passes understanding remains. Women in a personal relationship with Christ talked about the presence of hope in their lives.

Peter expressed the reality of that hope in 1 Peter 1:3–8:

Blessed be the God and Father of our Lord Jesus Christ, who according to His abundant mercy has begotten us again to a living hope through the resurrection of Jesus Christ from the dead, to an inheritance incorruptible and undefiled and that does not fade away, reserved in heaven for you, who are kept by the power of God through faith for salvation ready to be revealed in the last time. In this you greatly rejoice, though now for a little while, if need be, you have been grieved by various trials, that the genuineness of your faith, being much more precious than gold that perishes, though it is tested by fire, may be found to praise, honor, and glory at the revelation of Jesus Christ, whom having not seen you love.

Peace and Pain Coexist

When my first husband was killed, the inexpressible comfort of God seeped into all the hurting nooks and crannies of my life and lifted me above the circumstances. I remember trying to explain this spiritual reality to a friend who just couldn't understand. He thought that I meant I felt no pain as a result of God's presence in my life, even as he was watching me endure a great deal of pain.

I tried to tell him how pain and peace coexist. I felt tremendous loss and piercing pain at the same time that I rested confidently in the assurance that God would see us through that terrible time in our lives.

If relief during mid-life circumstances means only the complete absence of pain, we don't have the answer. But if relief means abundant life full of spiritual fulfillment that coexists with pain, we have the only authentic answer.

If relief for physiological symptoms of menopause means only the complete disappearance of the symptoms, we don't often have the answer. None of the women interviewed had hot flashes stop when they prayed in the middle of the flashes (although there may be some women who have experienced that kind of relief). But the relief that women did find was in the ability to handle the distress and discomfort of their symptoms.

Looking for Empowerment

Many of the secular books on menopause put a strong emphasis on self-empowerment. Some of this emphasis is in response to women being treated badly for centuries—sometimes in the name of Christ or the church.

Many women have felt degraded for all their lives. The idea of having power over themselves is a tempting enticement. In her book *Woman at the Edge of Two Worlds*, Lynn V. Andrews writes:

> In this book I work with four of my women apprentices in Los Angeles who are experiencing menopause in very diverse ways. Together we build new ways of empowering our lives and the lives of our families through new spiritual integration with our everyday world.[5]

Some of the suggestions in these secular books hold out great appeal to women who are seeking help.

Many women in the focus groups expressed frustration over years of being told what to do. Some grew up in homes where fathers were domineering. I as well grew up in a home dominated by an angry father. I learned that in order to survive I had to figure out what he wanted from me and try to meet those requirements. He wanted perfection and he wanted me to think like he did. When he couldn't control my belief in Jesus Christ, he seriously undermined my ability to believe that I could think for myself.

Other women in the focus groups sat under church leadership that discouraged any view but that of the leadership. Questioning was synonymous with heresy. Yet their questions may not be related to salvation as much as, Who am I as a woman before God? They felt pigeonholed by men who group women in categories that do not allow for individual expression or inquisitive thinking. These women were neither feminists nor men-haters. They were not, for the most part, angry. They were simply tired of feeling like they have mental limitations that distance them from God and who He wants them to be.

We talked in the groups about the struggle for Christian women to strike a balance between learning to be proactive on their own behalf and releasing control of their lives to the Lord. Many women feel weak because of other people telling them what to do instead of weak in recognition of their dependence on the Lord.

Jesus said, "My grace is sufficient for you, for My strength is made perfect in weakness" (2 Cor. 12:9). But Jesus did not say that the strength of someone other than Himself is to be made perfect in our weakness. When power is relinquished to Jesus, the result is gracious leading. When power is abused by others, the result is often ungodly control.

The Growth of Faith in Trial

The deep, personal faith in God that can emerge from the fires of mid-life frees women and releases them to experience the gracious goodness of acceptance by Jesus. This power of Jesus is exciting. It requires a new kind of relinquishment. It is not a relinquishment of self that annihilates individuality. It is a surrendering of self into the hands of a loving God who, in turn, encourages growth, welcomes questions, loves unconditionally, and expresses Himself through the surrendered.

The women in the focus groups expressed less fulfillment with rituals, like tightly-structured Bible studies, and more fulfillment in their relationships with the Lord based on much more personal encounters with Him. They are still reading their Bibles, praying, and going to church. But the essence of their contentment lies in their total openness with God, which results in knowing they are personally loved and accepted. They bring their doubts and questions to Him about true meaning and their place of value in His plan and are reaffirmed in their faith. They do not feel reprimanded for asking. They have not abandoned the doctrine of repentance for sin. In fact, there is much deeper repentance. But the repentance comes more as a result of hearts breaking over inadequately loving God and others than of focusing on the breaking of long lists of rules. There is less guilt over missing a church service and more concern about showing Christ's love to the world.

Self-empowerment Changed to Christ-empowerment

There is power in lives that are committed to Christ and surrendered to Him. This power results in an attitude of trust and security, for your interests are being cared for infinitely. There is contentment that God is in control even when we do not feel like He is. Empowerment does not rest on our limited abilities to make life happen as we wish. Empowerment rests with the God of creation.

The unbelieving world grasps at holding onto the reigns of life. While the teaching of self-empowerment holds great appeal, it falls short. Sooner or later, women realize that they really are powerless over so many aspects of their lives. They may be able to make choices that enhance their lives temporarily, but ultimately they don't have the wherewithal to stop hot flashes, or look twenty-five, or live forever.

And when they are finally faced with the question of death, they have nothing to compare with the reality of eternal life found in Christ.

CHAPTER 13

....

FACING MORTALITY

....

*T*he secular world has little to offer in answering the question of how to face death. Some people believe in reincarnation, some believe that death is simply the end of existing, and others don't know what to believe.

I was talking recently with a woman who is an atheist. She said, "I really don't care if I die and worms crawl in and out of my body."

I felt sad for her. If she really does believe that, she faces a dismal end. Her focus, and the focus of many women, is on living this life to the fullest at the present moment. It seems, though, that this viewpoint is harder to maintain as women age. It is one thing to focus on the present when there is a lot of the present remaining. It is another to focus on the present when you may be close to the end of your life.

That is one of the reasons why many menopausal women begin to think about death. The changes in their bodies during menopause clearly indicate that they do not have unlimited years ahead of them. They are in the second half of life—at best. The reality of death is the crucible in which the amazing Christian doctrine of eternal life rises victorious above all other beliefs about what happens after death.

Death is still an enemy to be endured, but for the person who has a personal relationship with Jesus Christ, immortality in heaven waits on the other side of death.

Behold, A Pale Horse

The book of Revelation is the account of the apostle John's look into the future. John depicts death starkly: "So I looked, and behold, a pale horse. And the name of him who sat on it was Death, and Hades followed with him" (6:8).

I have heard the hoofbeats of the pale horse many times. When I was ten years old, my grandmother lived with us. I loved her deeply. But one morning I was awakened before dawn by the arrival of the doctor and my cousin, Ron. My grandmother had had a cerebral hemorrhage in the middle of the night and was dying. As she lingered on in her bedroom, I watched other people arrive: the minister, my uncle, a few neighbors. No one spoke directly to me. They were busy, but I knew what was going on.

At nine A.M., my mother asked Ron to take me with him to the hospital to pick up a rubber sheet. We rode in silence on our errand (designed, I knew, to get me out of the house). As we were driving home, I remember sensing the moment she was gone. The sky turned slate gray and a damp mist hung heavily over the car as we crossed a bridge over the Brandywine River.

Nanny is gone, I said to myself.

I was cold. It was winter, but I was cold way down deep inside. Death is cold. When the pale horse comes, he breathes the frigid breath of the grave on those who watch him snatch life from the one they love. He rides off into the darkness leaving the pain of loneliness in the hearts of the living.

During the war in Vietnam, I heard the hoofbeats with frightening frequency. Calls in the middle of the night told my first husband and me that our friends had been ripped from life while fighting in a jungle far away. Several women I worked with lost husbands and loved ones. Military funerals became a part of life. Death was always close by. When he wasn't sweeping in to carry off someone we knew, the pale horse was stomping the frozen ground of my memory. The telephone was an enemy. Every ring held the potential for more grief.

I was a Christian when most of these young men left my life. But I was not around other Christians so I viewed death as the end. In my late twenties, my first husband, Jack, and I became active in an evangelical church that stressed the doctrine of eternal life. I changed from seeing death as only the end of life to seeing death as an end that led to a better beginning. Jack and I were gratefully enveloped in this reality of eternal life for about six years before the pale horse rode back in.

When Jack was killed, I heard the familiar hoofbeats again, but the deep, cold, dread of the past was gone. Death was still an enemy. Death still meant loneliness of heart. Death ripped my world apart in one dramatic swoosh of a hot-air balloon bashing into electrical wires and falling in flames.

But this time, the horseman on the pale horse was not the final victor.

> "O Death, where is your sting?
> O Hades, where is your victory?" (1 Cor. 15:55).

I knew the moment that Jack took his last breath he was in heaven. The loss was ours, the victory his. He was in a place of perfect peace. We would be together again. The Cross had overcome the grave and the horseman on the pale horse could only touch us this side of heaven.

The reality of heaven doesn't take away the pain of loss. But it gives indescribable hope. Life doesn't end. Not only does it last eternally, but it becomes a place of perfection instead of a place filled with pain.

Amazing Grace

Women in their mid-life years think about death. Many of us have been personally touched by the loss of a loved one. Many of us have already faced the invasiveness of disease. We have watched our friends receive news of illness and then endure treatment that devastates the quality of life. Despite the painful realities of aging, we as Christians have a hope that transcends even years of difficulty on earth.

I want to tell you about my friend, Ann Reed.

When I came to interview her, she was sitting on a swing in her front yard, smiling. She looked beautiful— for any age. Her big, brown eyes twinkled as she came across the lawn to hug me. I was amazed that this woman of beauty and grace was suffering the ravages of cancer.

Ann was sixty-seven years old at that time. When she was forty-two she had a hysterectomy. After the surgery, she was immediately given estrogen. Ann did not remember being given an option. Her doctor simply told her she would be on estrogen the rest of her life.

Ten years later she developed a malignant lump in her breast. After this surgery, she was taken off estrogen. She remembered the menopause symptoms raging full force—night sweats, mood swings. She begged for estrogen.

"I said I would risk cancer again if I could only have estrogen. That's when my doctor told me my cancer was probably estrogen-induced."

Her doctor told her that the surgery had removed all the cancer, allowing for an immediate breast implant. She had no chemotherapy or radiation, but the doctor refused to give her estrogen again.

Ann had no sign of any more trouble until October 1991. She was hurrying to answer the phone when she heard a bizarre sloshing sound inside her body. She went to the doctor thinking she had pneumonia, and her lung *was* retaining fluid. But when the doctors drained her lung, they found cancer cells. Further testing showed that the cancer had already spread from her lung to her liver. She began chemotherapy in January 1992. The treatment lasted for seven months. Then Ann was in remission.

The remission lasted about one year. When I interviewed Ann in August of 1993 she had just gone back on chemotherapy. She was due to go back in to the doctor to see if the therapy was working.

I asked Ann if any of her doctors had suggested a nutritional approach as treatment for her cancer, and she said they had not. Her doctors had agreed that there was no statistical proof that a nutritional approach would do any good.

Ann reaffirmed that her ultimate confidence is in the Lord.

"I was never angry. I never questioned, 'Why me?' 'Why now?' It is almost a settled condition that He is very aware and my confidence is in the fact that He is the Great Physician," she said with a peaceful expression.

I couldn't keep the tears back as she spoke.

"The reason I am so earthbound is because it's all we know. Heaven will be so wonderful but we don't know it experientially."

She told me that she and her husband, Kenny, have talked openly about the likelihood of her death. They know that they will long to be together again; knowing that they will ultimately be together keeps them from being morbid about it.

Six months after my first visit with Ann, I called for an update. That day I spoke to an excited woman.

Three weeks earlier her doctor had informed her that the chemotherapy was not producing any positive results, and had recommended that she simply enjoy life and call a hospice in a few months.

Shocked and discouraged, Ann turned to a different approach when she received a brochure publicizing a seminar given by Anne and David Frahm.

Anne Frahm had been pronounced a hopeless cancer case. She wrote of her recovery from cancer after traditional medical methods failed to help her. In the introduction to *A Cancer Battle Plan: Six Strategies for Beating Cancer from a Recovered "Hopeless Case,"* she writes:

> For a year and a half I read every book and underwent every conventional therapy—surgery, chemotherapy, radiation, and hormone therapy. Finally, presented as my last option, I underwent an autologous bone marrow transplant. When this, too, failed to send my cancer into remission, the medical world pronounced me "hopeless." Not ready to lie down and play dead, I turned elsewhere. Within five weeks after starting a strict program

of detoxification and diet under the guidance of a nutritional counselor, my cancer had packed its bags.[1]

My prayer for Ann was that she would have as miraculous a recovery as Anne Frahm has had. But that was
not to be. Ann slipped from this life into heaven on October 31, 1994. She lived and died with amazing grace.

And that's what it's all about: the amazing grace of
God poured out in the lives of those who invite Him in,
whether it's for the horror of cancer or the ongoing
stresses of menopause. We have help in living with pain
in the present with the hope of a dwelling place with no
pain in the future. The apostle John gives us another
image from the book of Revelation of that place:

> Now I saw a new heaven and a new earth, for the first
> heaven and the first earth had passed away. Also there
> was no more sea. Then I, John, saw the holy city, New
> Jerusalem, coming down out of heaven from God, pre-
> pared as a bride adorned for her husband. And I heard
> a loud voice from heaven saying, "Behold, the taberna-
> cle of God is with men, and He will dwell with them,
> and they shall be His people. God Himself will be with
> them and be their God. And God will wipe away every
> tear from their eyes; there shall be no more death, nor
> sorrow, nor crying. There shall be no more pain, for the
> former things have passed away" (Rev. 21:1–4).

New Beginnings

We all want to experience wholeness. We want to be
fulfilled in mind, body, and spirit. We want to be physically, emotionally, and spiritually healthy.

It is the spiritual component of our lives that pulls all
the other elements of healthy living together. Even in
the face of poor physical health we can experience full-

ness of life because our spirits have grasped the reality of living above and beyond the limitations of life this side of heaven.

Experiencing spiritual reality isn't easy. Physical and emotional pain are not insignificant interruptions to our lives. They can devastate us, thwarting our attempts to rise above our circumstances.

Menopause can be a trying time. It is a time of change and decision, and wholeness may seem elusive. Spiritual resources may seem far away in the face of debilitating symptoms and confusing choices. Even the most stalwart of religious women may find themselves perplexed at their inability to cope with life as they used to.

One woman, who has been in Christian leadership for many years, was experiencing hot flashes and emotional stress. Her doctor wasn't answering her questions to her satisfaction so she went to see a doctor recommended for his expertise in hormone therapy. When he spoke to her in a condescending manner, she cried all the way home in exasperation.

This woman is spiritually mature and highly adept at appropriating the means of grace in her life. Her faith has remained unshaken, but her usual calm in the midst of difficulty has been challenged since menopause arrived.

This time of life is a process. It is not a permanent destination. Time will pass, moments of calmness will increase, and the feelings of fragmentation will disappear. In the meantime, it is the spiritual component that keeps us as women moving forward. God is alive and operative on our behalf.

There is so much of life and opportunity still ahead. Wherever you are in the process of menopause you can study and choose from numerous options for treatment. You can strike out on a new path that interests you or pick up an old dream and give it life. You can drink from the spiritual waters that God pours out on your life and let those personal blessings spill over into the lives of your family and friends. You can change and grow and enjoy life to the fullest.

Pain and challenges will not disappear, but you can meet them with wisdom and grace. You can move from menopause to maturity feeling good about yourself and your future. You can experience life filled with excitement and hope.

So much is ahead. There are so many new beginnings.

APPENDIX

....

STARTING A SUPPORT GROUP

....

*T*he women I interviewed in the focus groups loved the experience of meeting and talking with other women about the specific topic of menopause. They appreciated hearing other women express feelings like their own with vulnerability and sincerity.

Some of these women have gone on to join or to start support groups. They are finding encouragement and help in making their own decisions about menopause and other issues that occur during mid-life. Most of all, they feel uplifted and hopeful. The groups are a safe place where they can identify with their peers and openly share all of their feelings.

If you are interested in joining a group, begin with your local newspaper under the section that lists group meetings open to the public. Or call your local hospital (ask for their women's section or ongoing education) and ask about a menopause support group.

Or you can start your own group.

Suggestions for Getting Started

1. Make a list of your friends between the ages of forty and fifty-five.
2. Call those you think may be interested in forming a menopause support group.
3. Schedule your first meeting solely for the purpose of discussing what the members of the group want most from a group.
4. Have the meeting in a private home, in a room where women can talk freely without the hostess' family members overhearing the conversation.
5. Agree to maintain confidentiality in the group.
6. Agree to accept the validity of various forms of treatment, so that women can be honest about what methods they are trying or thinking about trying.
7. Schedule the first several meeting times.

One Example of a New Group

A friend of mine started a support group recently, out of her own interest in hearing what other women are experiencing.

We met in Carol's home on a Tuesday morning. Some of the women work but have flexible schedules and were able to meet in the morning. There were seven of us for the first meeting.

As we didn't know everyone in the group, we spent most of the time just talking freely about where we are right now. It was a relaxed time of getting to know each other; we were all about the same age and experiencing similar symptoms.

We decided to meet once a month, to discuss information we may have discovered and to share how we feel and what choices we are making. Our group wanted to be able to talk freely and enjoy identification with other women who understand this time of life.

NOTES

Chapter 1: What Is Happening to Me?

1. Wulf H. Utian, M.D., Ph.D. and Ruth S. Jacobowitz, *Managing Your Menopause* (New York: A Fireside Book, 1992), pp. 58–59.
2. Lois W. Banner, *In Full Flower* (New York: Vintage Books, 1992), p. 273.
3. Ibid., p. 285.
4. Ibid., p. 274.
5. Ibid., p. 274.
6. Gayle Sand, *Is It Hot in Here or Is It Me?* (New York: HarperCollins Publishers, 1993), p. x.
7. Amanda Spake, "The Raging Hormone Debate," *Health*, January-February 1994, 47.
8. Susan Ince, "The new hormone therapies: Rx for Superwoman?" *Vogue*, September 1993, 384.

Chapter 2: Hot and Cold and All Shook Up

1. Dr. Sharon Sneed and Dr. David Sneed, *Prime Time* (Dallas: Word Publishing, 1989), p. 15.
2. Utian, p. 35.
3 Linda Ojeda, Ph.D., *Menopause Without Medicine* (Alameda, CA: Hunter House Inc., Publishers, 1992), p. 32.
4. Mary Beard, M.D. and Lindsay Curtis, M.D., *Menopause and the Years Ahead* (Tucson, AZ: Fisher Books, 1991), pp. 35–36.

5. Winnifred B. Cutler, Ph.D. and Celso-Ramon Garcia, M.D., *Menopause: A Guide for Women and Those Who Love Them* (New York: W. W. Norton & Company, 1992), p. 150.
6. Joe S. McIlhaney, Jr., M.D. with Susan Nethery, *1250 Health-Care Questions Women Ask* (Colorado Springs: Focus on the Family Publishing, 1992), p. 544.

Chapter 3: Where's My Mind and Where's My Waist?

1. Utian, p. 58.
2. Ibid., p. 100.
3. Raymond G. Burnett, M.D., *Menopause: All Your Questions Answered* (Chicago: Contemporary Books, Inc., 1987), p. 19.
4. Beard and Curtis, p. 5.

Chapter 4: Explaining the Controversy

1. Utian, p. 73.
2. Spake, p. 47.
3. Anne Louise Gittleman, *Super Nutrition for Menopause* (New York: Pocket Books, 1993), p. 9.
4. Leslie Vreeland, "Health dept. top causes of death," *Lear's*, March 1994, 41.
5. D'Arcy Fallon, "Food supplements battle is brewing," *Gazette Telegraph*, 29 August 1993, sec. B, p. 5.
6. Utian, p. 15–17.

Chapter 5: History of Hormone Replacement Therapy (HRT)

1. Robert A. Wilson, M.D., *Feminine Forever* (New York: M. Evans and Company, Inc., 1966), pp. 53–54.
2. Ibid., p. 116.
3. Ibid., p. 156.
4. Spake, p. 48.
5. Hershel Jick, M.D., Richard N. Watkins, M.D., Judith R. Hunter, Barbara J. Dinan, R. N., Sue Madsen, B. S., R. Ph., Kenneth J. Rothman, Dr. P. H., and Alexander M. Walker, M.D., M. P. H., "Replacement Estrogens

and Endometrial Cancer," *The New England Journal of Medicine* 122 (February 1, 1979): 220–221.

6. Cutler and Garcia, p. 121.
7. Lila E. Nachtigall, M.D. and Joan Rattner Heilman, *Estrogen: The Facts Can Change Your Life* (New York: Harper-Perennial, 1991), p. 4.
8. Cutler and Garcia, p. 175.
9. Utian, p. 90.
10. Gretchen Henkel, *Making the Estrogen Decision* (New York: Fawcett Columbine, 1992), p. 76.
11. Paula Dranov, *Estrogen: Is It Right for You?* (New York: A Fireside Book, 1993), p. 87.
12. *Premarin: What Every Woman Should Know About Estrogen*, prod. by Ayerst Laboratories Inc., New York, videocassette.
13. Dranov, p. 101.
14. David T. Felson, M.D., M. P. H., Yuquing Zhang, D. Sc., Marian T. Hannan, M. P. H., Douglas P. Kiel, M.D., M. P. H., Peter W. F. Wilson, M.D., and Jennifer J. Anderson, Ph.D., "The Effect of Postmenopausal Estrogen Therapy on Bone Density in Elderly Women," *The New England Journal of Medicine* 329 (October 14, 1993): 1141.
15. Marianne J. Legato, M.D. and Carol Colman, *The Female Heart* (New York: Avon Books, 1991), p. 29.
16. Ibid., p. xii.
17. Sandra Coney, *The Menopause Industry* (North Melbourne, Australia: Penguin, 1991), pp. 174–175.

Chapter 6: Begin Where You Are Now

1. Utian, p. 67.
2. Ibid., p. 68.
3. Legato, p. 29.
4. Nachtigall, p. 27.
5. Ojeda, p. 72.
6. Beard and Curtis, p. 33.
7. Utian, pp. 40–41.
8. Ojeda, pp. 58–59.

Chapter 8: I Don't Want to Read Another Word About Diet and Exercise!

1. Utian, pp. 108–110.
2. Utian, p. 118.

Chapter 9: Relaxation Breaks

1. Richard J. Foster, *Celebration of Discipline: The Path to Spiritual Growth* (New York: Harper & Row, Publishers, 1978), p. 15.
2. Florence Littauer, *Dare to Dream* (Dallas: Word Publishing, 1991), p. 43.
3. Julia Cameron, *The Artist's Way* (New York: Tarcher/ Perigee Books, 1992), p. 6.

Chapter 11: What Wives Wish Their Husbands Knew

1. Carol Henderson, "Divorce Over 55: The Bottom Line," *Woman's Day,* February 1, 1994, p. 23.

Chapter 12: Looking for Relief and Power

1. Barbara Ehrenreich, "Coming of Age," *Lear's,* September 1993, p. 45.
2. Sand, p. 132.
3. Gail Sheehy, *Silent Passage* (New York: Random House, 1992), p. 144.
4. Germaine Greer, *The Change: Women, Aging, and the Menopause* (New York: Alfred A. Knopf, 1992), p. 379.
5. Lynn V. Andrews, *Woman at the Edge of Two Worlds: The Spiritual Journey Through Menopause* (New York: Harper-Collins Publishers, 1993), p. 5.

Chapter 13: Facing Mortality

1. Anne E. Frahm with David J. Frahm, *A Cancer Battle Plan: Six Strategies for Beating Cancer from a Recovered "Hopeless Case"* (Colorado Springs: Pinon, 1992), p. 10.

BIBLIOGRAPHY

Beard, Mary, and Lindsay Curtis. *Menopause and the Years Ahead.* Tucson, AZ: Fisher Books, 1991.

Billingmeier, Shirley. *Inner Eating: How to Free Yourself Forever From the Tyranny of Food.* Nashville: Oliver Nelson Books, 1991.

Coney, Sandra. *The Menopause Industry: How the Medical Establishment Exploits Women.* Alameda, CA: Hunter House Inc., Publishers, 1994.

Cutler, Winnifred B., Ph.D., and Celso-Ramon Garcia, M.D. *Menopause: A Guide for Women and Those Who Love Them.* Rev. ed. New York: W. W. Norton & Company, 1992.

Diamond, Harvey, and Marilyn Diamond. *Fit for Life.* New York: Warner Books, Inc., 1985.

Dranov, Paula. *Estrogen: Is It Right for You?* New York: A Fireside Book, 1993.

Frahm, Anne E., with David J. Frahm. *A Cancer Battle Plan: Six Strategies for Beating Cancer from a Recovered "Hopeless Case."* Colorado Springs: Pinon Press, 1993.

Gittleman, Ann Louise. *Super Nutrition for Menopause.* New York: Pocket Books, 1993.

Henkel, Gretchen. *Making the Estrogen Decision.* New York: Fawcett Columbine, 1992.

Jenkins, Jerry B. *Winning at Losing.* Chicago: Moody Press, 1993.

Legato, Marianne J., M.D., and Carol Colman. *The Female Heart.* New York: Avon Books, 1991.

McIlhaney, Joe S., Jr., with Susan Nethery. *1250 Health-Care Questions Women Ask.* 2d ed. Colorado Springs: Focus on the Family Publishing, 1992.

Nachtigall, Lila E., M.D., and Joan Heilman. *Estrogen: The Facts Can Change Your Life.* Rev. ed. New York: Harper Perennial, 1991.

Ojeda, Linda, Ph.D., *Menopause Without Medicine: Feel Healthy, Look Younger, Live Longer.* Rev. ed. Alameda, CA: Hunter House Inc., Publishers, 1992.

Sand, Gayle. *Is It Hot in Here or Is It Me?* New York: Harper-Collins Publishers, Inc., 1993.

Sheehy, Gail. *Silent Passage.* New York: Random House, 1992.

Smith, John M., M.D. *Women and Doctors: A Physician's Explosive Account of Women's Medical Treatment—and Mistreatment—in America Today and What You Can Do About It.* New York: Dell Publishing, 1993.

Sneed, Sharon, M.D., and David Sneed, M.D. *Prime Time: A Complete Health Guide for Women 35–65.* Dallas: Word Publishing, 1989.

Utian, Wulf H., M.D., Ph.D., and Ruth S. Jacobowitz, *Managing Your Menopause.* New York: A Fireside Book, 1992.

*I*NDEX

heart disease, 48–49, 66–67, 70, 75–77, 81, 87
Henkel, Gretchen, 63–64
high blood pressure, 75, 76
hormone pills, 72
hormones, 3, 4, 39, 40, 49, 52, 85, 93, 145
hot flashes, 3, 17, 22, 26, 37, 43–44, 69, 145, 151
HRT (hormone replacement therapy), 22, 27, 33, 36, 40, 41, 42, 43,
    49, 51–52, 56, 57–68, 71–78, 81–87, 92, 145, 164
  risk factors in taking, 72–73
hypercholesterolemia, 73
hyperlipidemia, 73
hypertension, 73, 75, 76
hypoglycemia, 22, 77
hysterectomy, 8–9, 40, 51, 136, 160

In Full Flower (Banner), 8–9
Is It Hot in Here or Is It Me? (Sand), 13, 145

Jacobowitz, Ruth S., 6, 32, 34, 52, 63, 76, 98, 106
Journal of the American Medical Association, 54

kidney disease, 77
Kuller, Dr. Lewis, 64

lactose intolerant, 77
Lear's magazine, 54
Legato, Dr. Marianne J., 67, 73
Littauer, Florence, 119
liver disease, 72, 77

Making the Estrogen Decision (Henkel), 63–64
mammogram, 88, 91
Managing Your Menopause (Utian & Jacobowitz), 6, 34, 52, 72, 98
McIlhaney, Jr., Dr. Joe S., 28
memory loss, 32–34
menarche, 74
menopause (see subpoints)
  age, 6
  age at onset of, 1
  biblical view, 10–12
  changing attitudes, 13, 37
  dating during, 135–137
  definition, 1, 6
  fears associated with, xi, 3, 157–165
  historical attitudes toward, 8–9, 36, 42, 44
  late, 74